BREAST CANCER IN THE EIGHTEENTH CENTURY

STUDIES FOR THE INTERNATIONAL SOCIETY FOR CULTURAL HISTORY

Series Editors: *Anu Korhonen*
    Birgitta Svensson
Editorial Board: *Chris Dixon*

TITLES IN THIS SERIES

FORTHCOMING TITLES

www.pickeringchatto.com/isch

BREAST CANCER IN THE EIGHTEENTH CENTURY

BY

Marjo Kaartinen

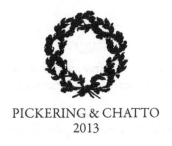

PICKERING & CHATTO
2013

Published by Pickering & Chatto (Publishers) Limited
21 Bloomsbury Way, London WC1A 2TH

2252 Ridge Road, Brookfield, Vermont 05036-9704, USA

www.pickeringchatto.com

© Pickering & Chatto (Publishers) Ltd 2013
© Marjo Kaartinen 2013

To the best of the Publisher's knowledge every effort has been made to contact
relevant copyright holders and to clear any relevant copyright issues.
Any omissions that come to their attention will be remedied in future editions.

BRITISH LIBRARY CATALOGUING IN PUBLICATION DATA

Kaartinen, Marjo, 1964–
Breast cancer in the eighteenth century. – (Studies for the International Society
for Cultural History)
1. Breast – Cancer – Patients – History – 18th century. 2. Medicine and psy-
chology – History – 18th century. I. Title II. Series
362.1'9699449'009033-dc23

ISBN-13: 9781848933644
e: 9781848933651

This publication is printed on acid-free paper that conforms to the American
National Standard for the Permanence of Paper for Printed Library Materials.

Typeset by Pickering & Chatto (Publishers) Limited
Printed and bound in the United Kingdom by the MPG Printgroup

CONTENTS

ACKNOWLEDGEMENTS

Through the years, a number of people have taken interest in my project: they have sent me notes on sources and patients, commented on my papers and ideas, read my manuscripts and helped in every possible way imaginable. I am grateful beyond words. My thanks go to Natalie Zemon Davis, Väinämö Nikkanen, Lauren Kassell, Laura Gowing, Tom Linkinen, Alexandra Lembert, Päivi Pahta, Eva Johanna Holmberg, Matti Rissanen, Wendy Churchill, Marika Räsänen, Miri Rubin, Sally M. Miller, Mary Beth Norton, Elaine Chalus, Kirsi Tuohela, Charlotte Merton, Anu Korhonen, Rita Hirst, Ellen Valle, Anne Laurence, Caroline Bowden, Sanna-Kaisa Tanskanen, Anne Summers, Deborah Simonton, Hanne Koivisto, Amy Erickson, Raija Vainio, Jinty Nelson, Natalie Bennett, Eero Perunka, Minna Nevala and my anonymous referees. There are some whom my thanks no longer reach: Patricia Crawford and Peg Keranen are greatly missed. I am in deep gratitude to Ellen Valle for correcting my English. Collectively, I would like to thank the editorial board of the series and everyone at Pickering & Chatto as well as everyone at the various conferences and seminars who have given me feedback, and I want to express my deepest gratitude and debt to my fantastic colleagues and students at the Department of Cultural History, University of Turku, and last but not least, all my wonderful friends and family.

Great thanks go to the University Libraries of Turku, Åbo Akademi, Cambridge and the University of California, Los Angeles, the Huntington Library, the British Library, the Wellcome Library, the (past) Wellcome Institute in London, and of course to my alma mater, the University of Turku.

Research for this book has been generously supported by the Academy of Finland.

PREFACE

Eighteenth-century breast cancer was a nightmarish, greatly feared disease. As a disease, cancer horrified people so much because of its slow and usually extremely painful progress towards a torturous death. Cancer in the breast[1] was considered the most common of cancers and the most dangerous: it seemed to kill with frightening certainty. Since antiquity, it had been thought that breast cancer was cancer *per se*; the breast was considered the most common location of cancer: an anonymous author wrote that when '[o]ne has a Cancer in any part besides, Twenty have them in their Breasts'.[2] Eighteenth-century authors have left us many suggestions relating to how common they thought the disease to be: it was considered 'frequent', and a surgeon further corroborated that '[i]f it were necessary, I could give an almost incredible Number of Instances, where such Circumstances have ensued'. Some considered London specifically. It was thought that breast cancer was common in London: 'in this over-grown metropolis there are great number affected in the same manner', and another surgeon testified that '[i]n London I have been consulted in many hundred cases'.[3]

While common, and even though cancer was in theory considered usually incurable, physicians, surgeons and other healers tried desperately to understand cancer and eagerly tested new medicines, and surgeons radically improved their operating techniques. Cancer was and had been a metaphor of many evils since ancient times, used to describe nearly anything seriously damaging, various phenomena that ate something alive.

Typically, cancer in the breast was immediately suspected and feared if a breast developed a peculiar lump or became painful; luckily, of course, many men and women were relieved to notice that these signs passed without any further trouble. The trouble was that much too often the first scare proved justified.

This book is about cancer in the breast in eighteenth-century Britain; it discusses the myriad ways in which this disease was understood, diagnosed and treated, and explores the ways in which those who had cancer or suspected to have cancer dealt with this illness. Regardless of the severity of cancer as well as the indescribable painfulness of premodern treatments, this book argues that the patients remained agents of their lives until the very end. They never gave up their right to make decisions concerning their own bodies. Finally, it looks at the emotional turmoil this gruel disease and its progress aroused in patients, their friends and families as well as their caretakers.

Sources

While as much emphasis is put on the sufferer's point of view as possible, it is the medical word that inevitably dominates eighteenth-century discussion on cancer. Few patients wrote about their experiences of cancer or their treatments. The famous account of Fanny Burney from the early nineteenth century is without a peer in the history of premodern mastectomy: no-one else described his or her experience in such detail and with such realism. This letter which Burney wrote to her sister nine months after her operation must thus be taken as an exception, and with a pinch of salt: while it is tempting to generalize about her experience, it is also risky to draw far reaching conclusions about one individual's and especially a professional author's experience of an operation. Regardless of its limitations, this letter is used in this work, of course, as are all the accounts I have been able to locate. Without doubt more personal patient evidence can and hopefully will be found in the future.

Some evidence of breast cancer comes from private letters and some from diaries but most of the evidence we can find of any individual suffering for instance comes indirectly from the patients' caretakers words: their physicians and surgeons' manuscript casebooks and various genres of publications. Eighteenth-century casebooks are, however, useful sources even if one looks at the patient's experience as their authors often used the patient's own accounts of their histories, if not verbatim, at least to a certain degree respecting their interpretations. This was important in making a diagnosis as well, and this thus adds to the 'authenticity', if one may, of the accounts in medical books.

The eighteenth century saw a tremendous flow of printed texts on various medical issues, and cancers were no exception. Thus a great number of medical treatises can be utilized when one wants to understand eighteenth-century diseases. The number of books that explain about cancer in the breast at least with a passing note rises to hundreds, and there are dozens of treatises that deal with this illness more extensively.

These medical treatises are not all written only for professionals of medicine. It must be remembered that in the eighteenth century professional medical discourse was still rather close to lay medical discourse. Same recipes were utilized, and medical books intended for the lay audience very much resemble the contents of the books intended for a more professional readership. The latter texts may be more direct and explain certain cancer processes in a more detailed manner but guidebooks for the layperson did not by any means censor knowledge on cancer, their progress or the sad fate it often brought.

While focusing on England and to some extent Scotland, it must always be remembered that medicine was highly international. From the seventeenth century onwards, it was quite usual for young men from the British Isles to study medicine abroad, especially Leiden.[4] Thus it was quite natural that medical books were eagerly translated into English to transmit and change ideas.[5] Quite a number of authoritative medical texts used in Britain were English translations from a number of languages, most obvious from French and German; some were translated from Latin but some minor languages such as Swedish can be found in the source material. To some extent these translations have been regarded here as English books as they were in the vernacular, meant for a large at least the general professional medical audience and they were an important part of eighteenth-century medical discourse in Britain.

In this medical discourse it still was typical in the eighteenth century to comment and even copy each other. At times, when a characterization is central to my argument, I may note these similarities within texts. As it is not the nature of this study to trace the histories of the ideas on cancer or to be a textual analysis, I have not attempted to trace all these chains of 'loans'. It is not important for my argument who was the first to write about a certain idea: it is more important to note that the idea existed at a certain point in history as it may help us understand the experiences of cancer.

This study is greatly indebted to the work of many great historians of medicine and culture. When trying to understand early modern medicine and the patients' experience, especially fruitful are the works of Barbara Duden, Andrew Wear, Michael Stolberg, Mary Fissell, Roy Porter, Margaret Pelling and many others. While early modern breast cancer has received relatively little scholarly attention, Daniel de Moulin's short introduction to the history of breast cancer remains authoritative. James Olson and others have addressed breast cancer in their studies on breast cancer but their focus has been on later times. This book is an attempt to describe eighteenth-century cancer in the breast and its treatments in fuller terms.

Editorial Note

Original spelling and punctuation has been maintained with the exception of 'vv', which has been modernized to 'w'.

Notes
1. I use the terms 'cancer in the breast' and 'breast cancer' alternately, being fully aware that breast cancer is a modern term.
2. Anon., *An Account of the Causes of Some Particular Rebellious Distempers Viz. the Scurvey, Cancers in Women's Breasts, &c.* ([London?], 1670), p. 23. The anonymous author refers here to Paulus Aegineta, a seventh-century Byzantine physician.

3.   In the quoted order: J. Aitken, *Principles of Midwifery, or Puerperal Medicine,* 2nd edn (Edinburgh, 1785), p. 24; R. Guy, *Practical Observations on Cancers and Disorders of the Breast, Explaining their Different Appearances and Events. To which are Added, One Hundred Cases, Successfully Treated Without Cutting* (London, [c. 1762]), footnote on p. 54; H. Fearon, *A Treatise on Cancers; with an Account of a New and Successful Method of Operating, Particularly in Cancers of the Breast or Testis,* 3rd edn (London, 1790), pp. 195–6; W. Rowley, *A Treatise on the Management of Female Breasts during Childbed; and Several New Observations on Cancerous Diseases,* 2nd edn (London, 1790), p. 76.

4.   R. O'Day, *The Professions in Early Modern England, 1450–1800: Servants of the Commonweal* (Harlow etc.: Longman, 2000), p. 231.

5.   C. Deshaies-Gendron, *Enquiries into the Nature, Knowledge, and Cure of Cancers ... Done Out of French* (London, 1701); P. Dionis, *A Course of Chirurgical Operations, Demonstrated in the Royal Garden at Paris,* 2nd edn (London, 1733).

1 'ONE OF THE MOST GRIEVOUS AND REBELLIOUS DISEASES': DEFINING, DIAGNOSING AND THE CAUSES OF CANCER

In the long eighteenth century, cancer was considered to be among the most horrible diseases, a misery which one could hardly wish for anyone:

Is there a Man you hate,
Or wish the hardest Fate,
Bid neither Plague, nor Pox,
Nor fam'd Pandora's Box,
Bid neither Gout, nor Stone,
But (letting these alone)
If wretcheder you'll make him,
Then bid the Cancer take him.[1]

In medical discourse cancer was characterized in intense terms: it was 'of all the maladies to which human nature is subjected, the most formidable in its appearance'; 'one of the most loathsome disorders to which the human body is subject'; 'miserable and deplorable'; 'the most grievous and rebellious', 'horrid' and 'cruel' disease, indeed 'one of the most excruciating and intractable maladies incident to human nature'.[2] William Nisbet elaborated on the horrors of cancer:

With a slow, but rooted grasp, it undermines the existence at a more advanced period of age, and under the torments of the most exquisite and lingering pain, as well as a state of the most loathsome putrefaction, it consigns its miserable victims to a late but long wished-for grave, after rendering them, by its ravages, even still more than the former malady [scrofula] hideous spectacles of deformity.[3]

John Aitken noted that even the slightest sign of cancer was a reason for examination of the situation: 'Cancer is always full of danger, the slightest degree of it is justly alarming.'[4] Benjamin Bell considered breast cancer especially threatening: 'A real cancer is perhaps the most formidable disease to which the human body is liab[le]: Wherever it is seated, its consequences are to be dreaded; but more especially when fixed on one or both of the mammae.'[5] *A Compendium of Physic* (1769) characterized cancer, a medical mystery, as the shame of physicians; it was 'perhaps, the most dreadful malady, to which the human body is subject; is justly called the opprobrium medicorum, as it bids defiance to every method yet attempted, for a radical, compleat cure'.[6] Henry Fearon wrote that 'our fellow creatures' who suffered from cancer were 'unremittingly tortured with this dreadful disease', and he noted that the disease was 'excruciating and loathsome'.[7] Thomas Frewen considered it 'the most terrible evil' that befell the body,[8] and in a similar vein Benjamin Gooch described it as 'the most formidable and deplorable disease that human nature is subject to'.[9]

Inevitably, physicians and surgeons putting an effort into curing this horrible disease deserved praise. Human misery caused by cancer is stressed in the declaration of a Society which set out to study the disease and to improve the condition of female cancer patients among the poor:

> In the long train of diseases to which human nature is subject, no one is attended with more hopeless misery than that which is denominated cancer, whatever part of the body may be the seat of it. This occurs far more frequently than is generally supposed; and a calamity so pitiable as that of persons afflicted with cancers, in any rank or situation in life (all being alike subject to them) it is hardly possible to imagine; their sufferings being aggravated by the present insufficiency of medicine, to afford any proportionate relief.[10]

Cancer was seen not only as cruel but devious as well. Lorenz Heister noted that the tumour could remain in a small state for a considerable period of time, but then suddenly become aggravated and increase dramatically in size.[11]

Cancer was often given such human attributes as it was thought of as a live beast – this was especially true before the eighteenth century,[12] but this idea can be found in eighteenth-century writings as well. When Daniel Turner turned in his book from the discussion of benign tumours to cancers, he put his rhetorical skills to use to create a dramatic shift. He emphasized the great horror that cancer often was met with: it was a beast, like a lion, deadly dangerous:

> But we hasten to the Cancer, which we so lately left as a Lion sleeping, whom finding now provok'd, and rousing up, we shall (however happening to be foil'd) prepare to encounter him the best we can.[13]

This lion was often provoked, and eighteenth-century healers of all sorts were faced with the ravages of the disease. Cancer of the breast was one of its many manifestations, and it is to this I now turn and focus on throughout the following work.

Defining Cancer

Eighteenth-century surgeons and physicians generally made a difference between a benign cyst which they often called schirrus (pl. schirri) and a cancerous tumour, but there were other ways of typology as well. Jean Astruc divided breast cancers into two different types. The first of these began life as 'a knot in the breast', which gradually grew into a cancer. The other was a cancer originating as a schirrhus, which 'occupies all the mammary body'; this again turned into cancer. Both types of breast cancer could be either occult, inward or ulcerous.[14] Pearson noted that '[a]ll Schirrhi have a tendency to terminate in Cancer',[15] an idea which most seem to have shared. Many also admitted that a precise diagnosis was very difficult. Scrofula for instance added to the difficulty, as it could affect both men's and women's breasts.[16] In general, however, I would like to argue that cancer in the breast was not an umbrella diagnosis for different breast problems; physicians and surgeons often had a very clear idea of what cancer was like, and were able to differentiate it from other kinds of breast illnesses.[17]

Laypersons too were considered to be able to recognize certain kind of growths as being cancerous. In recipe collections and medical self-help books distinction was made between different breast problems. *The Queens Closet Opened* (1659), for example, listed recipes for sore breasts, promising an excellent and certain cure for all sore 'paps' but did not promise to cure either cancer or fistula.[18] A specialist and a well-informed layperson could thus at least in theory assess the degree of malignity of a tumour by interpreting the patient's symptoms. The widely acknowledged Galenic signs of malignity, 'itching, heat, shooting pain, and sudden increase of the tumour',[19] remained much the same through the period studied here. Richard Guy formulated this in clear terms: schirrus was not painful, but cancer usually was.[20]

The signs of malignity were so vague that it was difficult to recognize the moment when the transformation from schirrus to cancer took place. More generally, however, the process of change could be seen and felt. Joseph Warner's sixty-four-year-old patient, E.W., had had a small tumour in her breast for seven years, giving only occasional 'pricking pains'. The tumour started to increase in size very rapidly, and in only eight months grew 'to a considerable size and extent'. It was then excised, with good success. Rapid growth of a tumour was a grave sign, and cause for immediate extirpation.[21]

There were other signs as well:

> An occult Cancer is known to be formed ... when, after the Signs of a preceding Schirrus, a Titillation, Itching, Heat, Redness, are gradually perceived; with a shooting, burning, pricking Pain. The Colour of the Skin likewise changes from a Carnation to a deep Red; then it becomes purple, blueish, Livid, and at length Black: The Part feels very hard, unequal and rough; then it rises with an Apex in the middle; the Swelling increases, and the adjacent Veins become tumid, knotty, varicous, thick and black.[22]

Benjamin Gooch admitted that it was very difficult to say at which precise point, which specific moment a tumour turned from benign to cancerous. He thought it best to immediately remove all tumours surgically in order to avoid future danger from the growth.[23] Gooch's suggestion is in line with the prevalent idea that any tumour was potentially hazardous, and could turn into cancer. Therefore any tumour was always bad news, and was often, as we shall see later in more detail, considered a death sentence.

Cancer could be diagnosed from its appearance. Following the ancient tradition it was believed to resemble a crab when it advanced in the breast. The tumour was surrounded by crossing dark veins which resembled the pincers and feet of a crab, and the eighteenth-century authors often reiterated this idea.[24] In reporting the appearance of a cancer case in 1815, Samuel Young considered this kind of characterization justified and logical:

> In the description of this tumour, the usual attendant characteristic of advanced Cancer, in the instance of large varicose veins, is not to be omitted. These vessels appear in a very marked degree of disease, rising from various parts out of the very substance of the tumour. They crawl down its sides in a tortuous course, affording that appearance of claws, whence, in particular, the ancient name has been attached to the disease.[25]

There was a tendency to consider a large tumour more malignant than a small one, or rather to assume that malignancy grew with the tumour, but for most authors a cancerous tumour could in practice be of almost any size, from the size of a pea, commonly mentioned as the size of the tumour when it was first discovered, to that of a melon or even a very large melon such as 'a pompion', which was the size of an adult's head.[26]

It seemed inevitable that in most malignant cases the patient would eventually suffer from ulceration of the tumour.[27] It is safe to assume that ulceration was considered common at the later stages because it made a diagnosis quite certain. Pearson pointed out that ulceration was at times very rapid and he called this kind of process very violent.[28] In fact, ulceration in advanced cases indeed was common: a systematic study of untreated breast cancer patients in the Middlesex Hospital between 1805 and 1933 shows that 68 per cent of the patients went into ulceration, a stage considered desperate.[29]

Bryan Cornwell analysed the process of ulceration as follows:

> The skin rendered thin by violent straining, is at last burst by the contained matter; hence the ulcer, which by the continuance of the same causes that produced it, increases. While the blood vessels remain unhurt, a ferous ichor only appears in the ulcer; but when they are corroded, blood also issues forth, and as the fungous flesh dissolves, some pus is generated. The stinking sanies is from the heat of the part, and the access of the air putrifying it.[30]

Ulceration almost became to mean a synonym for the last stage of the disease. According to Richard Brookes, cancer ran an inevitable course first towards ulceration and then, almost inevitably, death:

When it [the tumour] begins to break, the Skin is excoriated, and there transudes through it a thin, sharp Ichor.

After this the sound Vessels on the Edges of the Cancer, being distended by the rising of the Tumour, are broken; hence arises a Putrefaction, which, turns into a sub-tile, sharp, fetid, cadaverous Sanies, which, corroding and eating away the sound Parts, makes a Progress in Depth as well as in Circumference, and sends forth malignant Roots, by which it takes fast hold; the Lips become tumid, parched, and offensive to the Sight; the Pain is intolerable, with a Sense of burning, pricking and gnawing; the Colour becomes cineritious, livid and black. Afterwards arise occult Cancers communicating with the Glands; Hoemorrhages; Convulsions; a slow Fever; a general Wasting; Loss of Smell; callous Tubercles in the Ears without Pain; fainting Fits. The Parts being thus eaten away and consumed, Death ensues.[31]

Because of this inevitable link between ulceration and death, ulcerated cancers were in general terms not surgically removed until the second half of the eighteenth century. Surgery was considered beneficial only if the tumour was smallish. If it had already ulcerated it was considered too late to be curable, and only palliative treatment was to be applied.[32] The progress of the disease was admitted to vary greatly. Many patients suffered for years, whereas others would be dead in months.[33] According to the study of the Middlesex Hospital patients, the median time of survival after first signs of cancer was three years. Ten years after the first appearance of symptoms, only 4 per cent of the patients were still alive.[34]

Diagnosing Cancer

The diagnosis of breast cancer was made by sight, feel, touch, smell and, occasionally, taste.[35] Tasting the different excretions of the patient was not completely unheard of in the latter part of the eighteenth century.[36] Sometimes diagnoses were still made through letters, the physician not ever seeing the patient but in these cases the senses were exercised by someone who mediated: a husband, a friend or the patient herself. Sir Hans Sloane, for example, received an account of a tumour in the breast, for which he was supposed to formulate a diagnosis and a prescription; above the account are written in a different hand four questions, depicting the main points in recognizing a malignant tumour. The patient's representative then responded to these questions:

Whether the edges of the tumour are even or unequall.
If there be any constant pain or upon change of weather or in the night.
If there was any blow on the breast or formerly a milk sore.
If it be large.[37]

These answers were essential in making a diagnosis. As we saw earlier as well, the sharp pain caused by the tumour was considered a diagnostic tool.

My sources strongly suggest that British physicians and surgeons examined their patients with their hands if needed. Many a physician or surgeon reported feeling a lump being loose or liquid. Alexander Morgan noted: 'A maid of about 23 years of age, of a healthfull complexion, came to me complaining of a continuall pricking pain in her breste. I looked up on it & felt a hard gland of an oval figure moveable.'[38] Morgan clearly looked at the breast and felt it. Hence palpation was part of his diagnostic toolbox. John Hunter described the tumour of Mrs Farhill as being of 'the size of an Egg when I was consulted. *I found it* perfectly moveable in and on the surrounding parts: no thickness could be found leading to the sternum nor to the arm-pit, nor any swelling in the glands of the arm-pit.'[39] Had he been making these remarks from what he was told, most likely he would have written that the tumour was moveable and that there was no swelling of the glands. Indeed, my research indicates that even vaginal examination took place.[40]

All these examples speak a different story from that of the case in Germany. Barbara Duden has argued for a 'taboo against touching the body'.[41] German doctors such as Storch carried out autopsies on some patients, but when the patient was alive they would not examine them by touching their bodies – in fact Duden argued there was no need to touch: one could read from the outside signs about the state of the body inside.[42] Touching was not a taboo on the British Isles even though the patient's permission was needed, but as I will argue later, it was indeed the patient who actively sought help and probably did not want to refuse palpation if that was considered necessary. It is perfectly possible, however, that the period witnessed a transitory phase in medical practice. It is entirely plausible that surgeons had always used their hands to examine their patients, their domain being external to the body, with its ailments, tumours, ulcers and wounds, while physicians would have kept to their ancient skills of diagnosis, largely concerned with the internal workings of the body. At a time when the medical fields of physician and surgeon were separate, the physician's practice would not necessarily have derived much benefit from a manual examination of the patient, which may well have created a taboo towards the patient's body, especially towards touching it, and probably also seeing the most intimate parts as well.

Diagnosing a breast cancer could not be an exact science; there was always an element of uncertainty. This was resolved by patience. One had to wait and see what the breast would do, what would happen with time and with mild treatments and diet: either the breast would soon prove cancerous, or the patient would be cured. This is what happened to a gentlewoman who developed a very sore breast which broke during her lying-in: she had to wait. The breast became so painful and runny, resembling a 'fistulous cancer', that cancer was a reasonable fear. Bathing and the use of liniments and English pills to purge her inwardly cured her in sixteen weeks, and the threat of cancer was revoked.[43]

Full diagnosis required careful consideration of signs: was there pain involved, and if so what kind of pain? Was there a growth of 'fungous flesh'? What was the nature of the humour discharging from it? It was especially important to understand the patient's medical history, to ask about the origin of the disease, whether it was outward or inward, to know if the patient still had her menses or not and if the patient was otherwise healthy or not. It was especially important to know if she suffered – or had suffered earlier – from 'the scurvy, scrophula, or venereal disease'. These were interrelated and could all turn into cancers. And, finally, in fact, the woman's body type mattered: 'the thin and bilious' fared better than 'those who are fat or full of blood'.[44]

Causes: Blockages

The causes of cancer puzzled eighteenth-century minds. There was a consensus that one way or another obstructions were formed in the body, and these obstructions caused tumours which then in certain circumstances could turn cancerous.[45] Theories abounded as to how these obstructions were caused, but the basic idea of the origin of cancer was similar in different schools of thought. In most theories the birth of cancer was attributed to different humours, fluids or juices, sometimes even 'viruses'. In Galenic medicine cancer had mainly been understood to be caused by the black bile, the 'blacke choler', which was concentrated – or 'superabounded' – in a certain place:[46] 'as in the face, eies, eares, but especially in such, which are more loose, spungye, full of kernels, receiuing naturally the grossest matter of blacke choler, as are the nostrells, lips, and breasts. But it is most vsually incident to the matrice and breasts in women.'[47] The case was even worse if the melancholy was extremely thick or black, since thick fluid was more prone to concentration.[48] Once this concentration had taken place, the melancholy in this spot became putrefied and formed heat. The patient often felt this as pain: it would now 'ake and burne'.[49]

This tradition lived on towards the eighteenth century regardless of the fact that Galenic theory had been more or less rejected in the seventeenth century. It was a logical theory and made sense according to everyday experience and examples of the tradition abound. For example, in 1700, David Irish advertised his pills against all kinds of illnesses, including cancers in the breast, caused by blockages especially in the liver, and relied heavily on the ancients.[50] John Moyle attested that cancer arose from acidity in the melancholy humour.[51]

Many eighteenth-century theorists thought that cancer was caused by other fluids. In 1713, Boulton, clearly reflecting new ideas but which never deviated very far from earlier theories, argued that cancer was born out of matter formed from 'Crudites impregnated with the pancreatic [ju]ice, which, for want of being digested to its natural Pitch, is a crude acid, and so comes nearer [to?] the Nature of an austere, for which Reason we call it acid-austere'. This juice alone was not enough to cause cancer: it still needed the melancholic and choleric humours to acquire its hot and sharp nature.[52] It followed that people with melancholy temperaments were most subject to the disease; people of other temperaments were prone to it if their diet added black bile to their system or if they lived in a melancholy place.[53] The idea of lymph as the source of cancer rather than black bile or the melancholic humour had been supported by iatrochemical and iatrophysical theorists since the seventeenth century. In practice, again, these explanations held much in common; sometimes bile and lymph were thought to have a combined effect.[54]

Tumours were thus born out of masses of melancholic humour, poisons or nervous liquids. Whatever the theory behind the birth of the tumour, the block-age growing out of a tumour always had a reason to form, and there were various causes. In 1670, an anonymous author concluded as follows:

> A Cancer is as much as to a Crab, and is a hard painful Tumour, either Whole or Ulcerous, and is said to have its rise from many Causes; some say from ill Diet, Meat or ill Juice, or a hot quality, and thick and glutinous substance, and that Onions, Leeks, Garlick, Venison and hot Spic'd Meats, eat too plentifully, and hot fiery Liquors, that burn and make adust the Blood and Humours, such as Brandy, strong Wines, &c. immoderately drank, breed them. Others, that the Air, pertubations of the Mind, Melancholly, ill Habits of Body, hot, sharp Humours, where there is a discrassys of the Blood and Lympha, being fill'd with an Acrimonious Salt, and a malign Sulphur is their occasion. Others, that they seldom proceed but from Blows, Strokes, Punches, or such external Violence, ill handling, Tumours from curdled Milk upon Lyings in, Imposthumes, &c. by which means there being an acid Ferment in the Blood, or it may be Obstructions of the Terans, or some other illness, which oftentimes causes Humours to slow thither, where coagulating, is capable to produce a Cancerous Ger-men, especially upon ill management, so as in time it increases and arrives to to [*sic*] that degree of inveteracy, which we somtimes find them to be.[55]

The causes were so many that one could say that having breasts at all was the greatest risk of contracting cancer.

Risks

Being Female and Having Breasts

Both women and men had breasts but as *Bibliotheca anatomica* (1711) noted 'they don't rise high in Men, because they have scarce any Glandules; but in Women, they swell into a roundish Figure'.[56] This anatomical difference made the great difference in the probability of getting cancer in the breast in men and women. The locations of men's cancers were mostly 'the tongue, mouth, or penis', whereas in women it most often found its seat in the breast or uterus.[57] The greater number of 'glandules' in women's breasts made women more prone to cancer, but of course women in general were considered more prone to illness.[58]

In Galenic theory cancer was often considered largely a women's disease, one which affected their feminine parts, the breasts and womb.[59] Furthermore, it was thought that a cured breast cancer could re-emerge as another cancer, this time in the womb.[60] If the womb was the source of all evils, the curse was that the breasts received these evils from the womb since the womb and breasts were considered connected. When the Rev. John Ward and Mr Eedes opened[61] the body of Mrs Townshend, who had died of breast cancer in 1666, they considered her cancer to have been more or less local; but in his diary Mr Ward confirmed that Dr Needham had seen a string, 'a mamillary vein' stretching from the breasts to the womb.[62] These strings could also be called 'veins'.[63] Since antiquity the idea had prevailed that the female reproductive organs were thus connected to the woman's upper body: Helen King points out that 'the major anatomical feature distinguishing women from men is the existence of a *hodos*, a route extending from the orifices of the head to the vagina'.[64] Both ends of the *hodos* were open, and each influenced the other: when a woman had her menses, for example, her throat would hurt.[65] In *The Manuall of Anatomy*, Read maintained that a mother's milk was produced in the uterus.[66] The connection itself, that is the 'Sympathy or consent betwixt the womb and paps, so frequently observed in women',[67] was recognized and considered commonplace knowledge, but how this connection between the womb and the breasts was created remained a mystery. The consensus on the existence of this cord slowly began to dissipate from the seventeenth century onwards, but the idea lived on in many forms. Walter Charleton for example denied such constructions, but was ready to admit that there was a 'Chyliferous vessel' that would transport matter both ways.[68]

John Ball attested in his *The Female Physician* (1770), intended for a female readership, that cancer was mostly a women's ailment regardless of the fact that it was common in both sexes: 'as it generally attacks women, and more especially their breasts (sometimes the womb, &c.) I have thought proper to consider it in this place as their distemper, though not altogether peculiar to them.'[69]

Fearon too considered it a given that women were more prone to cancer than men, but interestingly he could not form an opinion as for the reason for this:

> Women are more subject to it than men: whether, on account of their constitutions being weaker, or because the parts distinguishing them from our sex, viz. the breasts, uterus, &c. are more extensive, or on account of the changes that their constitution undergoes, which renders it unfit for generation, I cannot take upon me to give an opinion.[70]

Women were constantly seen as the weaker vessels, and their weakness came in many forms. *The Modern Family Physician* (1775) informed its readers that women contracted cancer more often than men because they had more 'gross habits of body', and perhaps more emotional a nature as well, since the author identified 'violent agitations of the mind' as a common cause of cancer.[71]

No one gendered cancer more clearly than Henry Fearon: 'the parts that distinguish the sexes, and all other glandular parts, both external and internal in both sexes, are more subject to it [cancer] than any other part'.[72] For him, the very markers of the sexes determined the location of illness.

Richard Guy among others further attested that cancer in the breast was more dangerous than other cancers; it was 'attended' with more 'mischievous Consequences', and that one of the reasons breasts were the favourite seat of cancer was that they were 'most liable to suffer outward Injuries'.[73]

In their general anatomy breasts in men and women differed little. Jean Astruc came to note that male breasts had a similar anatomy to women's breasts but were only rarely used:

> In the breasts, besides these lymphatic veins, which are in continual and constant use, both in women and men, there are other particular vessels which should be described. They are never of any use in men; and only on particular occasions, in women: that is to say, when they give suck. These vessels are the lactiferous ducts; called so because they convey the milk to the nipple in suckling.[74]

Even though male breasts might in some views lactate, the whitish matter produced by them had since Aristotle been denied as having any nutritional value.[75] Lactating men were no more wondrous than menstruating men who now and then appear in medical books.[76] This slight difference was not enough to save men from getting cancer in the breast.[77]

In today's world the probability of a man to get breast cancer is 1 in 1,000; there is no reason to assume it would have been more common in the past. I have found few cases in which breast cancer was suspected in a man. Robert Bayfield recorded a case of male breast cancer in his *Enchiridion medicum* (1655). It was not a particularly dramatic case:

> A neer kinsman of mine was (eight yeavs agone) troubled with a cancerous tumour in his brest; for a certain time I bathed the part affected with *Oleum rosarum omphacinum*, & applied many plasters of *Diacalcitheos*, and it pleased the Lord to cure him. Yea (and contrary to the Aphorisme of Hippocrates) he lived many yeares after.[78]

Richard Guy recorded one male case in his book, and referred to another in Heister's surgery. Male breast cancer seems to have been new to him when he saw his patient Mr Thomas Maynard; indeed, he added a footnote to Heister's case in order to lend credulity to his own observations. Maynard had cancer in his left breast, which had been caused – we shall soon see that this is not uncommon – by a bruise ten years ago. Guy treated him for nine months, after which the patient returned home, cured.[79] Melmoth Guy's book included two male cases.

The first was that of a young boy, 'a lad about the age of sixteen', the son of a Mrs Evans. He had a small tumour in his right breast. Guy considered the tumour so small that he could easily try some of his resolvents, since if they failed to destroy the tumour, he wrote, 'I could at any time extirpate the lump by my remedy'. The boy was cured, however, without the caustic methods held in reserve.[80]

The other patient had trouble in his upper body, although probably not in the area of the breast; I mention it here anyway. He was a servant named John Ayther, who suffered from a 'cancerous fungus' and ulceration on his sternum, on the upper part of the pectoral muscle and near the tendon of the mastoid muscle. Ayther had been treated by another surgeon for a long time, with little help, but Guy was able to resolve his matter.[81] These two cases were listed in a matter-of-fact style; even the first one, which clearly mentioned that the tumour was in the breast, did not specifically contemplate the nature of the disease.

Somewhat more informative is the case of a Rev. Mr T—s W—e, found in Dominiceti's *Medical Anecdotes* (1781). His case history started with a scorbutic eruption, which he was advised to treat by travelling to the seaside to cure it with sea bathing. He travelled to Margate, only to grow worse: he 'had not been there three weeks, when, beside being seized with a head-ache, and a shortness of breath, a kernel made its appearance on the nipple of the left breast'.[82] The kernel grew rapidly, and during his stay in Margate it erupted, yet the sore eventually healed. The patient returned home, but

> he had hardly arrived, when, tormented with a perpetual itching of the *cicatrix*, he incautiously scratched it. An ulcer being thereby formed, he was advised to apply plaisters of Turner's-cerat to it, by the surgeon of his parish; who, in examining the sore, about a fortnight after, found the discharge had become ichorous. Mr. W—e accordingly repaired the better advice to London; where, having applied to Mr. S—e, he was immediately put under a slight *salivation*. In nine weeks, nevertheless, a *confirmed cancer* spread itself from the *mamella*, which had been the original seat of the complaint, to the *sternum*; and, to remove it, it was proposed to have recourse to the *knife*.[83]

Treating a confirmed cancer by salivation, that is with mercury, was not unusual at the time, but the proposal of an operation is interesting indeed. There seems in fact to be no difference whatsoever in this case compared to women's breast cancers. The tumour first appears on the nipple, then occupies the breast, and moves elsewhere as well, as was understood to be customary in cancers. The author saw the patient in time to be able to prevent what he considered a fruitless and cruel operation, and he proclaimed that he had cured the patient with his mild medications.[84]

Cessation of the Menses

A healthy body had natural flows. Amenorrhea was an immense danger because ample menstruation kept women healthy.[85] As the Hippocratic texts already confirmed, the ancient belief was that breast cancer was associated with the menopause – as was, for example, women's gout.[86] Blocked evacuations, in particular the menstrual flow, caused a high risk of cancer. Because of this, age was an additional risk factor: early modern writers usually recognized forty-five to fifty as the age of the highest risk for breast cancer,[87] suggesting that this was the age when most women reached amenorrhea. They spoke of the suppression of the menses; the term menopause was not in use. Women were thus especially susceptible to cancer of the breast but so too were men whose tumours were caused by changes in their haemorrhoids, in which case the causes of the changes themselves had similarly to be immediately removed, by regular phlebotomies for example.[88]

Pierre Dionis noted that out of twenty women afflicted with cancer, fifteen were between forty-five and fifty years of age.[89] James Latta went so far as to argue that he had never seen a true cancer in a younger woman's breast. All his women patients younger than thirty-six with tumours in their breast he had been able to cure with 'a gentle mercurial friction'. He was horrified that some of these women had been advised by other surgeons to have mastectomies.[90]

Henry Fearon also supported the idea that amenorrhea at that age was a danger, noting that the woman's constitution would indeed undergo changes at that time, leading to 'a strong tendency to produce cancer'.[91] Writing for a general audience, Sir John Hill discreetly spoke of the sudden ceasing of 'a certain discharge' being dangerous.[92] Pearson suggested not only that cancer was often a menace to women whose 'Catamenia cease to appear', but that cancer of the uterus was specifically a great threat to women whose menses had earlier been 'in a large quantity'.[93] Even though this period of life was risky, it was also a point, Tissot declared, where a woman's life could take a forceful turn:

> it also frequently happens, that their constitutions alter for the better, after this critical time of life; their fibres grow stronger; they find themselves sensibly more hearty and hardy; many former slight infirmities disappear, and they enjoy a healthy and happy old age. I have known several who threw away their spectacles at the age of fifty-two or fifty-three, which they had used five or six years before.[94]

In humoral theory, it was originally important to open up another route for fluids to take if the menses were suppressed. That the menses as such were less important than the possibility of some form of purgation is illustrated by the following case: a young lady from Wiltshire, Miss Clarke, had her tumour extirpated, and returned home well. Her surgeon, Richard Guy, proposed putting an issue on her breast to keep the fluids running. She refused, but in just weeks her menstruation became irregular and then ceased altogether. The breast grew worse; to ease the situation 'an Opening' then had to be made, and presently a teacupful of clear liquid issued from it. Miss Clarke's menses did not return, but the opening was kept in order for nature to work its course.[95]

Richard Nayler's view of this female 'crisis' was quite pessimistic, and he considered it a period of the gravest danger:

> The great caution required at that particular crisis is well known to the sex, and to every medical practitioner; for it is then when some important changes, either of a salutary or morbid tendency, are wrought in the female constitution. Either nature effects her purpose in a lenient and favourable manner, or the latent seeds of some disease are ripened into maturity, and some chronic malady is established, which either cuts short the patient's existence, or makes it painful to her; and happy is she, if Providence avert from her the lingering afflictions of a cancerous affection of the breast or uterus.[96]

In eighteenth-century terms, age was a separate matter. It was related to amennorhea, as we saw, but it was dangerous in itself.[97] In 1806, Richard Carmichael explained that 'every writer' since antiquity had noted that old age and barrenness indeed made one subject to cancer.[98] The parts affected with cancer were considered naturally low in vitality which the circulation of the blood would have brought to them; the parts further lost their vitality if they were no longer in use. The breasts, uteruses and ovaries of women and the testes of ageing men were thus most prone to cancer.[99] William Buchan offered a clear timeline: the greatest risk factor was, again, passing the threshold of forty-five years of age.[100] The slower nature of older persons brought benefits as well. Interestingly, Richard Guy noted that young people at an age at which 'Nature is vigorous' had to be especially careful with schirrus, since their tumours should always be considered an imminent danger, while in older people schirri could well remain dormant for years.[101] In terms of facility of cure, it was easier to cure those who were of a lively disposition than those who were more of the broody sort: 'the Dull, Melancholy, P[e]evish, and Passionate, are more difficult to be relieved, than the Lively, Chearful, Easy, and Placid'.[102]

Even though at high risk, breast cancer was not thought of as a disease of middle-aged women only. It was understood that it could attack a child as well, and a number of the cases discussed in this book will deal with women who were of child-bearing age. There were not many children diagnosed with breast cancer, but in early modern thought such a scenario was considered possible. A treatise on children's illnesses in general, in a chapter dealing with scrofula, noted that some medications against the disease could cause cancers, even mortal ones, including cancers in the breasts.[103] Hinting at the dangers of puberty, Bryan Cornwell noted, referring to Hollerius, 'that girls are subject to glandulous tumours whose menstrual discharges are scanty'.[104] Thus women of all ages were prone to cancer. It was a constant danger: not necessarily probable in any particular case, but always present as a threat. And the list of risk factors did not end there.

The Problem of Breastfeeding

Early modern women and men were acutely aware of the risks of childbed for a woman. Even a normal course of birth was risky and trying for the body, and various complications, fevers and inflammations were also a constant threat. Breastfeeding was sometimes considered the ultimate feminine experience,[105] sometimes recommended because it gave pleasure to the mother: 'There is a sympathetic connection between breasts and the womb; as the breast is tickled, the womb is aroused and feels a pleasurable titillation, since that little tip of the breast is very sensitive because of nerves that end there.'[106] Breasts were this way linked to the main issues of midwifery[107] – some but not nearly all authors on midwifery commented for example on cancer in the breast.

In the eighteenth century there were two camps, very much divided about the virtues of breastfeeding. Some felt that it was not necessary or even proper; for some it was the most natural thing to do. In public discourse the dangers of curdled milk to the mother received much attention; often it is impossible to say which was considered more dangerous, to breastfeed or not. Sometimes breastfeeding was seen as dangerous because the milk could form abscesses that were a risk of cancer, and milk would draw dangerous substances to breasts;[108] sometimes not breastfeeding was considered more dangerous because the rise of the milk had to be stopped, which could cause blockages. Either way there were dangers, and schools of thought were divided. Breastfeeding, along with motherhood in general, was a political issue;[109] but perhaps we should not make too much of it in relation to cancer in the breast.

Breasts mattered. William Rowley considered childbed the main cause of breast cancer. He thought that breasts were neglected in childbed; when the women became older, between the ages of thirty-six and fifty, the results of this neglect were manifested in the form of cancer.[110] The way this happened was as follows:

> When these vessels are over-filled, and the natural discharge through the nipple not encouraged, either by the child's sucking, or by any artificial means, then do the symptoms often prove troublesome, and are succeeded by violent pain, inflammation, excoriation of the nipples, abscess and induration. If this last be neglected in the beginning, it lays the foundation of the cancer, and in a number of years often degenerates into that dreadful disorder.[111]

During the eighteenth century breastfeeding became more fashionable amongst the elites. Lady Mary Coke noted in her journal in 1768 that the lady-in-waiting Lady Louisa Clayton had 'suckled her child', and evidence of this had been given to Lady Mary by Princess Amelia herself. But there was a problem with Lady

Louisa Clayton: Lady Mary was told by Madame de Viry that Lady Louisa Clayton had 'a cancer'. The journal notes that she hoped it was not true, and thought that Lady Louisa only had some less threatening condition, as she was or had recently been in childbed: 'complaints in the breast are common after lying in, & I fancy it may be some trifling disorder that is magnified into a cancer'. Lady Mary was indeed hopeful – no doubt it was common to exaggerate the dangers of breast complaints as women were so very afraid of cancer – the 'terrible distemper', to use Lady Mary Coke's words.[112]

Elizabeth Bar of Henlow, Bedfordshire thought that the tumour in her left breast, which had been there for six years, had 'originated from cold, and from the pressure of stays whilst suckling'.[113] Cold was dangerous for a breastfeeding mother, and there were advice books exhorting women to give up stays altogether as they were dangerous – and could even cause cancer itself.

As noted, it was not wholly unusual to think that breast cancer arose out of curdled milk in the breast.[114] Fanny Burney probably blamed this for her breast cancer since she had been forced to wean her son Alexander – 'What that has cost me!' she later exclaimed – when she developed an abscess in her breast two weeks after he was born. She later evidently held this as the reason for her renewed breast problems, which eventually led to her mastectomy.[115] There was a sixteen-year gap between these two occasions, since Alex was born in 1794 and her tumour emerged in 1810. Her breast problems had returned, and we have to take into account that her breast had been troubled several times before the tumour. In 1804, when Alexander was ten, she again had breast trouble, and wrote to her father in England: 'I am but just recovered from a very strong menace of inflamation [sic] upon the breast, but which has yielded to strict fasting & asses milk.' In November 1806 she wrote to her sister that she had 'just recovered from a Breast attack'.[116] Whatever this attack meant, we know for certain that she had had a long history of breast scares.

There was an understanding that milk abscesses or breast inflammations could turn into cancers, if not carefully treated.[117] Jean Astruc saw 'the collection of thick milk' as the premier cause of all tumours. Over time, if the compressed milk had an effect on the neighbouring parts, there was the risk of a harmless schirrhus turning into a true danger, cancer.[118] The causes that could make the milk move dangerously were above all the following: 'by a fever; the improper use of an acrid, saline, or heating diet; the use of too strong solvents employed imprudently to resolve a schirrhus; want of sleep; violent passion; the habit of drinking strong liquors or coffee'.[119] This is interesting because it was fundamentally the person's life choices that determined whether or not a tumour would grow.

Benjamin Bell also believed that untreated and especially wrongly treated breast inflammations caused by milk would in the worst cases lead to cancer.[120] He recommended plentiful bleeding, a good quantity at a time, as a good treatment, along with a cooling diet.[121] John Burrows strongly argued for the now fashionable necessity of breastfeeding, on the grounds that keeping the milk flowing prevented milk blockages and thus cancers:

> These obstructions are common to women who use that blameable practice of repelling the breastmilk to prevent suckling.
>
> I am sensible, that it is no easy matter to persuade some mothers to suckle their own children: however, it is incumbent on us to use our endeavours to induce them to perform this important duty, where it is not inconsistent which some present disorder. But if natural affection, and the innumerable inconveniences to which the mother exposes her child by refusing to suckle it, are not prevalent to do this indispensible duty; let her but consider, that by changing the natural course of her milk, she draws upon herself many diseases; such as abscesses, schirrous, and cancerous tumours, which are worse than any thing that can possible happen to her by suckling her children.[122]

Burrows tried to create guilt in mothers who decided not to breastfeed, and insisted that by their stubbornness they even 'drew' disease upon themselves. Richard Nayler was quite clear in his opinion that women who chose not to breastfeed their babies put themselves at risk of 'indurations of breast', which easily turned cancerous. His point is political and in favour of breastfeeding. There was no good way of extracting milk from the breasts other than giving suck: 'perhaps, there is no means of avoiding the possible bad consequences of a retention of the coagulated milk equal to the natural one of giving suck; a practice, to which it is equally the duty and interest of every mother to conform'.[123] All in all, this was in accordance with the general cultural idea that it was necessary and healthy to keep the different bodily fluids flowing.

Childlessness

As previously mentioned above, not giving birth, either by choice or infertility (the early modern term would be barrenness) and celibacy were considered major causes of breast cancer. This notion was again in accordance with the Hippocratic writers, according to whom 'if women have intercourse, they are more healthy'.[124] In France, de Moulin notes, the proportion of nuns in case histories was remarkable;[125] this is corroborated by contemporary evidence from Lorenz Heister[126] and from Pierre Dionis. The latter had travelled in France and wrote that nuns were at great risk: 'the disease was very rife in nunneries', he noted, and pointed out that almost all the patients had their menses suppressed.[127] In Britain Benjamin Gooch referred to Dionis's findings, but took no clear stand on the matter, but William Buchan was convinced that barrenness and celibacy were risk factors.[128] Bryan Cornwell too noted that celibacy constituted the strongest possible risk for cancer:

Celibacy, as well as the cessation of the menses, conduces to the production of cancers in women, whence antiquated maids are the most subject to them: next to these are those mothers who have not suckled their children; then those women who are past child bearing; and the least so are men, and those women who have bore children, and nursed them with their own milk.[129]

Sometimes discrepant voices were heard. James Nooth doubted that celibacy or barrenness were real causes of cancer in women. He duly noted that it was common to believe that cancers were especially typical of aged, childless women, but observed that schirrous tumours in fact often occurred in younger women who were still menstruating.[130]

Mechanical Causes

When explanations were sought for the origin of a tumour, mechanical irritation was a popular and sensible explanation.[131] Both doctors and patients were unanimous on the subject of mechanical causes as the possible reason for a cancer, and patients were frequently able to ascribe the history of their tumours to some accident or other mechanical cause. Not many doubted the possibility of cancer arising out of mechanical blockages. Among the few dissenters was Henry Fearon. He recognized the potential danger of external injuries, but was not convinced that a blow alone, for example, could cause cancer. He rather thought that perhaps a 'natural predisposition' was needed for the cancer to grow from an injury.[132] As said, Fearon's view is an exception to the rule; in the minds of most writers, external explanations were perfectly valid.

One very common explanation for a cancer in the breast was a blow received to the breast.[133] The blow had often been received years earlier, but was vividly recalled when the breast began to give worrying signs. At times there was a lump in the breast lasting for years, which then suddenly became painful.[134] De Moulin has noted that in the late seventeenth and eighteenth century, the French in particular seem to have been convinced that breast cancer would follow from sexual pleasure women received through their breasts.[135] I have not come across this concern in British sources, but feminine vanity does appear, in the form of tightly laced stays, and is sometimes blamed as a possible cause of breast cancer. Wiseman advised patients who had swollen glands in their breasts to 'avoid the lacing her self too streight [sic]', and cut 'the stiffening out of her Bodice'.[136] William Buchan and many others noted that among the causes of cancer were the friction and pressure women endured because of their stays: they squeezed and compressed the breasts, and occasioned great mischief.[137] Sir John Hill warned women whose breasts were already at risk of cancer to avoid tight stays.[138] In 1800 Anthony Florian Madinger Willich argued, in a book intended for the whole family, that nine out of ten women still used stays simply because their mothers and grandmothers had done so even though the practice was out of date and out of fashion. He claimed that 'cancer itself' might ensue if women did not give up such folly and prefer the 'Grecian form'.[139] However, I have come across only one actual case, that of the approximately twenty-eight-year-old Mrs Brownless treated by Guy, in which there was a suspicion that a cancer in the breast might have been partly due to her use of stays.[140]

Passions

From ancient times it was understood that passions such as sorrow, grief or anger could cause illnesses such as cancer; passions had the power to coagulate the humours, thus forming lumps.[141] The dangers of passions were recognized in the eighteenth century as well. Wiseman accounted passions as the cause of death of one of his patients. Her breast remained much the same for a considerable time, but then her husband died and other misfortunes followed: her menses ceased and her breast swelled. She died half a year later, having refused the knife.[142] Passions were not the sole cause of her death, as her menses stopped as well, but they were an important link in the causal chain Wiseman considered logical.

According to Bryan Cornwell, '[s]orrow, and other disturbance in the mind, easily converts a scirrhus into a cancer'.[143] William Falconer noted that it was understood that at least half of human diseases 'originate from the influence of passions on the human system'.[144] Grief in particular was a great danger.[145] Willich noted that grief was born out of sorrow, if it lasted long and was very great, but there were also stronger forms of sorrow: distraction, despair and agony.[146] Potentially deadly, continued grief could influence different parts of the body and lead to death through cancer – or even more quickly, through a broken heart.[147] In the same vein, Buchan listed the passionate risk factors: 'It may likewise be occasioned by excessive grief, fear, anger, religious melancholy, or one of the depressing passions.'[148] Henry Fearon who, as we have seen, was in general very sceptical about all explanations given for the origin of cancer, recognized the connection between the affections of the mind and the disease, but was reserved as to whether passions were effects or causes.[149]

Moving towards the nineteenth century, in 1815, John Rodman proposed that it was the woman's mind, always prone to hysterics, that caused breast cancer. Their heads were in any case weaker in every sense.[150] In eighteenth-century treatises, hysterics and delicate constitutions were characteristic of noble ladies. Richard Guy's cases for example make it manifest that those whom he mentioned as 'subject to nervous and hysterical Complaints' were members of polite society.[151] Members of all classes could get cancer in the breast; yet the causes were to some extent class related.

Inherited or Contracted Cancer?

John Peyrilhe concluded that it was impossible for cancer to be hereditary but others were more open to the possibility of cancer being a hereditary disease.[152] William Buchan for example included 'hereditary disposition' in his list of causes for cancer.[153] Between 1780 and 1781, Charles Bissett recorded his patient cases, among them including a young woman, a servant from near Helmsley. She had two ulcers; Bissett noted that there was reason to consider the possibility of cancer because the young woman's mother had died of a cancer in her breast.[154] When Arthur Nicolson, M.D. wrote a letter to a colleague describing a cancer in a forty-four-year-old lady's breast, he considered it worth mentioning that 'some of her family have died of cancer'.[155] His decision to mention this fact suggests that he considered it plausible that cancer was hereditary.

Henry Fearon, who was also sceptical about external irritation as a possible cause of cancer, noted that cancer was often considered hereditary, but that he found this difficult to agree with. In 1790, when he wrote his *Treatise on Cancers*, he had not quite made up his mind on the matter.[156] William Nisbet seems to have considered hereditary cancer self-evident; he notes that hereditary types progress more rapidly than those arising from outward causes.[157] John Pearson considered heredity to be one of the seven main causes of cancer.[158] Interestingly, William Rowley's *Seventy Four Select Cases* includes one in which he had prescribed medicine to prevent a recurrence of the disease because the woman had in his opinion a hereditary tendency to develop cancer: 'there has been a hereditary cancerous and schrophulous complaint in the family'. He prescribed medication to be taken twice a year, for six weeks in spring and autumn.[159]

Many more authors, however, commented on the contagiousness of cancer than on its possibly hereditary nature. Was cancer indeed a contagious disease? Quite a number of early modern scientists thought so,[160] and Peyrilhe, who doubted it was hereditary, experimented its contagiousness on a dog. He made a small wound on the dog's back, and with a syringe procured two drachms of the cancer fluid into the wound. He then covered the wound with 'a plaster and bandage'. He let it lie for three days; after opening it, he reported some ulceration, and 'a disagreeable smell'. Two more days, and the effect was even more 'violent': 'The whole skin, from the head to the tail, was compleatly emphysematous ... A little ichorous, blackish matter flowed from the wound.'[161] The dog suffered, but – to the relief of the modern reader – the test ended abruptly at the hands of his maid:

> The eyes of the animal were vivid, and he seemed to have great thirst: in this state the poor creature was perpetually howling ... [A]t length my maid, disgusted by the stench of the ulcer, and softened by the cries of the animal, put an end to his life, and thus prevented my observing the ultimate effects of this disease.[162]

Nicholas Tulp (Tulpius) supported the idea of contagiousness, and following him, so did many others. In fact there was little evidence to support the idea, but there was some, and it was thought important. In some places cancer patients were not allowed in to hospitals because of the fear they might transmit the horrible disease.[163] This of course suggests that cancer may have been considered something similar to leprosy – a devastating disease which would utterly destroy and consume the sufferer and endanger people around the patient. But it did not implicate the moral connotations carried by leprosy, which as David Nirenberg notes, was 'a disease of the soul, brought on by moral corruption and sin'.[164] Nowhere have I encountered the idea of cancer carrying similar meanings.

De Moulin suggests that the notion of the contagiousness of cancer was based on a single case, namely Tulp's patient, named Adriana Lamberta, who had suffered from an ulcerated cancer and who had conveyed the disease to her maid. De Moulin argues that it was this one case that kept the idea alive in Europe until the nineteenth century;[165] but in fact, British physicians and surgeons had native cases supporting the supposition. In Britain, Tulp's case did not customarily end up in medical treatises, but local cases recurred in a number of treatises.[166] One dissenter was John Pearson, who commented very critically on Tulp's findings. He noted that whereas Tulp claimed to have himself contracted cancer in his throat, the ulcers could not have been cancerous. Pearson claimed that '[s]urgeons and their attendants, expose themselves almost every day to the noxious effects of cancerous sores with perfect impunity; from whence it may be safely concluded, that the danger of infection is so small, as not to form an object of serious attention'.[167]

Among the influential local cases was that of Mr Samuel Smith, whose narrative I have located in five treatises with a timespan of more than a hundred years;[168] it is also mentioned in passing and anonymously in two others. In the latter part of the seventeenth century, Samuel Smith was one of the surgeons at St Thomas's Hospital in Southwark. His fate was quite extraordinary. He tasted 'the Juice, or Matter contain'd in one of the little Cystis's or Glands' of a large amputated cancerous breast. This he did to determine the nature of the juice, but it happened at great expense: it led, in his own opinion, to the consumption which took his life a few months after the experiment.[169] It was only natural for Smith to consider the juice of a cancerous breast highly poisonous, since it was widely considered to be sharp and corrosive. Thomas Willis, his contemporary, noted that 'Cancrous, Scrophulous, and Pestilential Ulcers, shew a most sharp humor, by which the flesh and Membranes are eaten, as it were with Aqua fortis, with a blackness poured on them'.[170] James Latta, a surgeon, also suggested that because of its corrosive nature the fluid was 'capable of infecting an healthy body with the same disease'.[171]

Ideas about the corrosive nature of the juice were fortified by accounts which spread widely. The surgeon William Beckett reported that he had read about a curious case that had taken place in New England: the husband had sucked his wife's sore breast to get rid of the cancerous poison, and had consequently lost all his teeth. Beckett did not believe that the explanation lay in the corrosiveness of the substance; if this were true, the husband would have harmed his 'tender Parts as the Gums, Lips, and Tongue' as well.[172]

It should be noted that the author of *An Account* did not speak of contagion: he merely considered the juice of the cancerous breast so poisonous that it was enough to kill Smith. But this of course left the door open for other contagions if one came in contact with the juice. In a similar vein, Beckett did not consider the point of the narrative to be contagion as such. Nor did he believe that the reason for Smith's horrible fate – Beckett in fact mentions that he was 'a Martyr to the Art of Surgery'[173] – was the corrosiveness of the juice (whether acid or alkaline, an ongoing debate). He rather found the reason for Smith's demise to be in 'the extraordinary Stench and Malignity of the Matter, which impressing its Virulency on the Animal Juices most undoubtedly disturb their regular Motions, and cause the utmost Confusion of the whole Æconomy'.[174]

Beckett's scepticism was based on his own experience. He said that news of Smith's manner of death 'did not a little surprize me, because I had several times had the Curiosity to do the very same Thing' – and for that matter in the same hospital. Beckett explained that he had often tasted the cancerous juice, first diluting it in several spoonfuls of water, until he tasted the juice proper.[175] This had not harmed him in any way.

Beckett argued for the possibility, although rare, of indirect contagion.[176] As an example of the abounding stories, he repeated one from Nottingham: a wife had cancer in her breast, and the husband, out of compassion, tried to relieve her suffering by trying to suck the matter out of her nipple:

> her Husband was of Opinion he cou'd relieve her by sucking it; accordingly he put this Method in Practice, in hopes without doubt he cou'd detect a Cure, by drawing the Cancerous Matter out of the Nipple; he continu'd his Attempts for some Time, but found it did not answer his Design; for tho' a small Quantity of Matter was discharged this way, the Disease still became worse, and she terminated her Life soon after. Two Months were scarce expir'd before the Husband of the Deceased came up to London, upon Account of a swelling he had arose on the Inside of the upper Jaw; he apply'd himself to some ingenious Surgeons for Advice, who assured him he must undergo the drawing of several Teeth on that Side of the Jaw which was affected, and have the Swelling, and Part of the Jaw-Bone (if necessary) cut away.[177]

Beckett also noted that a foreign surgeon had told him the story of a poor mother who had breast cancer and had shared her bed with her two small daughters. The five-year-old developed a painful tumour in her breast. The idea of contagion was based on the fact that the girl's breast was always positioned in the bed so that she was 'disposed to rub against the Dressings soaked in matter'. The mother, he decided, was not very diligent in changing them. The mother died, and so did the five-year-old, but the other girl remained well. For Beckett the explanation was not that the matter killed the girl; rather, he thought it remotely possible that 'the corrupted Fluid has attain'd an exalted Pitch of Malignity, to communicate some of its more active Particles to the Blood and Spirits; and so causing a very great Disorder in their Motions produce a violent Feaver, and Confusion of the whole Oeconomy so as to occasion a Person's Death'.[178]

Another case showed that cancer could be caused by coming into contact with cancerous substances, as happened to a three-year-old girl when she accidentally imbibed some of the liquid issued from an ulcerated breast. The case was one of Benjamin Gooch's; it was quite well known, and was used, for example, by the Scots surgeon James Latta as evidence of cancer not being merely a local disease,[179] while it was deemed incredible by John Pearson.[180] Gooch wrote that in 1752 he was asked to go to Norwich to see 'a person of great virtue and tenacity', a nearly sixty-year-old woman who had a cancerous tumour in her breast and an affected arm. Her story was quite exceptional, and clearly made an impact on Gooch. When she had been about three years old she went with her mother to see a friend who suffered from an ulcerated cancer in her breast. The ulcer had just been dressed, and there was a tea-cup on the table containing 'some of the liquor with which it had been washed'. The little girl accidentally drank some of it. Two weeks later an 'eating ulcer seized her tongue and one side of her mouth ... making dismal ravage of the cheek, as well on the outside as the inside'; the London surgeon who treated her found it very difficult to heal. He was successful, however, and it was twenty years before she next suffered from the effects of that accidental imbibing of the liquid: an angry abscess developing on her leg. Fifteen years after that she found a tumour in her breast, which grew slowly until she reached menopause. The tumour was now aggravated, grew more rapidly, and in the following years occupied her whole breast. The breast never ulcerated, but she died some time after Gooch had seen her.[181]

The case of this unfortunate woman, doomed because of an accident as a young child, speaks not only of the idea that cancer could be caused by contact with cancerous substances (which can be seen as contagion), but also about the fact that illnesses had very long histories: they had meanings beyond their own day, reaching in this case nearly sixty years into the past.

2 'BUT SAD RESOURCES': TREATING CANCER IN THE EIGHTEENTH CENTURY

As the eighteenth century drew to a close, cancer had to be declared 'absolutely incurable'.[1] The number of hopefuls and optimists who believed there were effectual remedies for cancer was always relatively low, and there is reason to suggest that towards the end of the century, following a period of great enthusiasm for substances such as hemlock, there were many who suffered from an intellectual hangover. The number of those who believed in the greater effectiveness of the knife seems to have been somewhat higher. Regardless of this slight disillusionment with progress, however, early modern people were and remained resourceful. In every generation, many physicians and surgeons were desperate to find ways to help their patients. It was one's duty to make an effort to hinder the development of the disease, according to one's profession, whether by extirpation or amputation or by mitigating the symptoms with a multitude of drugs available in the apothecary's shop, even if one admitted that these methods were 'but sad resources'.[2] It is striking how passionately eighteenth-century authors wrote about cancer and the lack of means to help their suffering patients.

In the following chapter, I take a look at these 'sad resources', from 'lean diets' to the scalpel; in other words, from palliative medicine to the physicians' pharmacopoeia, and thence in conclusion to the surgeons' craft. The direction is from mild towards what were considered radical treatments. The direction is also away from the familiar experience of the layperson: such a person was perfectly able to understand what kind of diet was good for her condition and to treat herself with various medications, as well as to make many of her own, but if she wanted to turn to surgical treatment she was much more dependent on the medical profession. This said, it must be kept in mind that surgical procedures were by no means monopolized by the surgeon.

Whatever the treatment chosen, palliative medicine was to some extent always in use: it was not only used to improving the (dying) patient's quality of life, but also to prepare the patient for any operation that might be carried out, and to assist her recovery from such an operation.[3] I first take a look at palliative methods, which in humoral theory and practice aimed at achieving a suitable humoral balance in the patient's body; when humoral theory was set aside (which was not always the case during the period under scrutiny here), palliative methods were used, for example, to pacify the irritating fluids of the patient's lymphatic system. I then move on to specific cancer medications; as we shall see, increasing emphasis was placed on the new medicines which from the seventeenth century onwards were being introduced into cancer medicine, especially by 'chemists'.

As I have suggested, there was great eagerness and optimism in the growing field of medicine particularly during the eighteenth century, and among the growing group of medical practitioners in the British Isles as well as elsewhere in the Western world, to find a cure for cancer in general and for cancer in the breast in particular. Along with new medications, such as hemlock and arsenic, other new forms of treatments were tested. Particular emphasis was placed on discovering a relatively painless and safe cure; thus, for example, the virtues of electricity and air for breast cancer patients were tried. None of the habitual forms of surgery were painless or safe – a fact which the proponents of surgery as the only possible cure for cancer saw as their worst enemy.[4] The eighteenth century witnessed the amalgamation of the professions of physician and surgeon: surgery became an academic field, and increasing effort was put into researching surgical methods and outcomes.[5]

Palliative Medicine

First, let us return to palliative medicine. It was, as mentioned above, overarching, affecting all patients whether they relied more on self-help or on a physician's care. Before any surgical operation, the patient purged her body and changed her diet to one more suitable. The principles of palliative medicine were universally familiar by virtue of necessity: one's health depended on everyday decisions which balanced the body by enjoying in moderation food and liquids, fresh air and warmth, exercise and rest. It was thus also understood by everyone that if a person became ill then it was expedient for them to make changes to their lifestyle. This was of course a matter of wealth and leisure: for those who could afford any excess in the first place, the ideal of moderation regarding food and drink was now tempered into abstemiousness, as one withdrew into the bed-chamber and avoided any strenuous movement. For the great majority of early modern people, however, this was an unthinkable luxury.

Lifestyle decisions mattered. A lump in the breast was a discovery requiring immediate action, and arguably everyone – whether determined on surgical removal of the tumour or aiming at palliative treatment only – believed that regulating one's diet was necessary. An abstemious lifestyle, i.e. limiting one's intake of strong foods and drink, was beneficial for a body showing signs of wavering balance. In practice one needed to consume substances that would not (in Galenic theory) heat or (in Helmontian theory) irritate the system. This meant giving up red meat, strong spices, great amounts of salt and any alcohol except mild wine, and replacing these with smaller portions and with milder, cooler foodstuffs. This was termed a lean and mild diet, a palliative remedy; it could not save a cancer patient's life, but could gain her several extra years than if she continued to adhere to excess in sweets, liquors and strong, salty meat.[6] As said, abstemiousness was envisaged as necessary for all patients throughout the early modern period. Writing at the end of the eighteenth century, the surgeon John Pearson summed up the importance of abstemiousness: 'without the strictest adherence to temperance no remedies whatever will prove efficacious'.[7] This meant that the patient was at least partly responsible for the outcome of her treatment, and that by taking an active attitude towards one's illness one could achieve more than by neglecting oneself.

Andrew Wear observes that early modern ideas on diet were long based on ancient ideals, and that the foundations of thought on the maintenance of health in general changed very slowly.[8] The principles of Galenic causation gradually disappeared in the writings of physicians and surgeons, but much of the content remained.

A typical Galenic cancer diet would suit most eighteenth-century practitioners. Crab meat was one such foodstuff.[9] Eating crab meat was thoroughly Galenic in nature: it would counterbalance the effects of the disease – which, as we recall, was in its essence a crab. Below I quote John Ball, who in the latter part of the eighteenth century recommends crayfish broth as part of a favourable cancer diet; this time arguably included in his list because crayfish was understood to be suitably 'soft good nourishment',[10] not because of the crab-like nature of the disease.

Because of its similarly excellent softness, milk was often mentioned, as in Textor, as a highly favourable foodstuff against cancer. A great number (if not in fact all) physicians and surgeons favoured a milk diet, especially one of ass's milk, oftentimes perceived to be especially soft and beneficial; to an extent that some writers promised that under favourable conditions it would cure cancers.[11] Among the advocates of milk was John Ball. In advising ladies as to how to treat themselves if they were troubled with a tumour, he suggested the following palliative diet (which, as noted, includes crayfish broth):

> [T]he aliment ought to be such as may afford soft good nourishment, as new-laid eggs, chickens, pullets, rabbets, mutton, veal, lamb, kid &c., and these boiled sometimes with barley, oatmeal, rice, millet, spinage, endive, succory, lettuce, sorrel, turneps and the like, are much better than roasted. To these may be properly added, at different times, asses, goats or cows milk, chocolate, cray-fish broth, viper broth, small welfleet oysters, harthorn jelly, millet, rice or light bread puddings, &c. carefully avoiding all manner of salt and high seasoned meats, pork, ducks, geese, cheese, and the like viscous food.[12]

His recommendations suggest that for Ball the importance of easy digestion is decisive. The focus is no longer on the humoralist notion of maintaining the balance of humours: what is now important is avoiding too much acidity.[13] While the end result of this favourable cancer diet tends towards softness and mildness, the reasoning behind this suggestion is no longer based on bodily balance but instead on digestion. Soft food was thus understood to be preferably cooked, not roasted, and to consist of mild vegetables, fresh ingredients, and of the meat of young animals, which promised that it would be tender. We also see the previous century's novelty and eighteenth-century great favourite, chocolate, among the aliments considered good for the digestive system.

While there was a certain consensus on the nature of a beneficial diet for cancer, there were also some individual opinions which stood out as exceptional and perhaps as experimental. Henry Manning's patients, for example, were recommended vegetarian diets; he wrote that cancer patients should not have any 'animal food'. As far as I am aware, he was the only doctor of his time to suggest this. He seems to have considered himself progressive and pioneering in proposing vegetarianism for this purpose, as suggested by the title of his book, *Modern Improvements in the Practice of Surgery* (1780). The basic idea behind his cancer diet was nevertheless similar to that of his colleagues, and along with vegetarianism his diet too was based on milk.[14]

In addition to a suitable diet, a patient was also expected to use similar prudence in the control of emotions; all excess was life-threatening. Hippocrates himself was mobilized to instruct readers that the cancer patient needed to remain in a calm and trouble-free state: 'a continual serenity, which springs from a good conscience, is, of all the affections of the mind, the greatest contributor to perfect health'.[15] Suitable happiness was brought on by having a good conscience, but it was also essential to eliminate destructive emotions from one's mind and replace them with more positive ones. One should avoid, it was duly noted, 'all manner of anxiety, grief, anger, or any other irregular passions of the mind', and gradually substitute 'others more agreeable in their place, such as mirth, gaiety and chearfulness'.[16] 'Continual serenity' was recommended; unsuitably large doses of positive emotions, such as 'mirth, gaiety and chearfulness', were also considered dangerous, as was all excess. Admittedly, this was true of all situations in life, moderation being a fundamental early modern principle.

The body thus moderated could maintain its favourable balance and stop the destruction due to illness by regular purges. In Galenic theory this helped reinstate the body's humoural balance, keeping at bay the tumour and the black bile which it formed.[17] Frequent purges were recommended for example by Culpeper; some of his colleagues even recommended that they occur daily.[18] In particular phlebotomy, bleeding, was considered so advantageous that it remained popular – and fashionable – throughout the eighteenth century, despite the Helmontians' vigorous declaration that purging was harmful and barbarous.[19] Various methods were in use. Wallis recommended a combination of bleeding and leeches,[20] while Ball suggested cupping or perhaps even an issue in the arm or leg if the patient's menses had been suppressed. In menstruating patients bleeding was less important, and more emphasis was put on vomiting and regular stools. These were ensured by 'gentle mild purgatives of manna and cream of tartar, dissolved in whey, or the purging mineral waters of Acton, Epsom, &c.'[21]

Waters were a fashion of the eighteenth century. 'Glastonbury water' was advertised for its promising effects, as having cured a difficult breast problem. Mary Crease, a miner's wife, had an old, extremely painful tumour in her breast, and took the water both inwardly and outwardly to rinse the breast. The water cured her.[22] In 1750 Richard Russell promoted sea-water for healing diseases of the glands, and made it popular, for both drinking and bathing.[23] It should thus not be surprising to find a lady sea-bathing in an attempt to cure her ills. An unnamed forty-year-old lady treated her tumour with sea-bathing, and it was reported that '[s]he bathed in the sea for three or four summers with sensible benefit; but during the course of the sea-bathing in June 1769, the pains in the right breast grew more violent, when she discovered a hardness in it, and the skin seemd contracted, without any discolouration; for which reason she gave up the bathing'.[24] This lady's use of sea-water was methodical; it was apparently used not only as a purge but as a soothing medication, and was probably taken as a course, with the hope of curing her tumour. This links sea-water to a long list of cancer medications, at which we now take a more detailed look.

Cancer Pharmacopoeia

Anyone diagnosed with cancer in the breast made an attempt to treat it. Early modern physicians and patients were determined to relieve the symptoms of cancer, pain and ulceration especially, and to find a cure for the disease. The role of the patient in determining her treatment is the focus of Chapter 3 of this book; suffice it therefore at this point to note that everyone used medications of some sort, that some were more eager than others to experiment, but that everyone was desperate to try something.[25] In addition to following a lean diet and regular purges, cancer patients took medicines well proven useful and helpful by generations before, new substances promoted by the chemists and the occasional sensational novelty promising to perform miracles.

Before going further, certain important points should be kept in mind regarding the treatments discussed here. First, and particularly with regard to treatments, there was no strict line between lay and professional (academic) medicine. Not only did many medical advice books written by professional physicians disseminate up-to-date information on illnesses and their cures for the use of a lay audience, but medicine itself was immersed in ancient knowledge which in many respects was already shared knowledge. Further, many physicians took into account what we would call women's knowledge, their recipes and cures for illnesses such as cancer. These recipes were widely used, and understood from experience to be beneficial.

Secondly, tradition was being only slowly undermined by specialization and professionalization of medicine. To some extent, the often reiterated shift in the eighteenth century towards an emphasis on academic medicine applied to cancer treatments. An early sign of this general trend was elite women's abandonment of their distilling houses by the end of the seventeenth century. Whereas up to then it had been the lady's duty to prepare medicines and act as a healer in her household, she now gradually placed increasing faith in apothecaries and university-trained men. This does not mean that she abandoned her recipe collection completely, but it does suggest a slow but definite shift towards professionalization in the whole field of medicine. Part of this professionalization, as already noted, was the amalgamation of the surgeon's craft with the physician's profession.

Theories of treatment abounded, and the number of medications used was thus also high. This is no wonder; cancer was a disease which fell into the territory of both surgeon and physician, understood to have both internal and external origins. N. D. Jewson famously attributed the wealth of theories and the consequent lack of thorough medical analysis to the physicians' social relationship with their upper-class patients. He argued that physicians as individuals were set on pleasing their customers in order to retain them. Pleasing a patient was best done if one could offer a cure. According to Jewson, it followed that physicians were not interested in the illness itself but in the cure of their patient.[26] While this proposition is somewhat undermined by the extensive early modern discussion on the nature of the cancer, as well as by the many practitioners who felt a deep and passionate need to find a solution to cancer, it effectively reminds us of the way in which cancer, like all disease, was treated: much emphasis, much hope was placed in novelties. As it was so clearly understood that there was no successful cure for the disease, the attitude towards new ideas was welcoming and research into cancer was regarded as important in many hospitals. Taking a different perspective from that of Jewson, and following Coates, the eighteenth century saw an important change: illnesses were beginning to be perceived as entities separate from the patient. The search was now for a cure for the illness, not the patient.[27]

Above, however, I have referred several times to traditional medicines. I take a brief look at women's own recipes in Chapter 3; here it suffices to stress the wealth of choice available. Both university medicine and medical advice books offered similar treatments. The ancient provenance of a cure was often mentioned to gain respectability for the advice: Boëthius, for example, had recommended limestone or Aqua Calcis for cancers,[28] as had his followers, while Pliny had advocated lettuce with saltpetre, pimpernels, mandragoras and especially betony (which he mentions as sovereign) for cancerous ulcers.[29] Along with ancient advice, ideas as to the virtues of more everyday plants were cultivated as well: for example, in the sixteenth and seventeenth centuries, buckwheat (backwheat or binacorne), petum and fluellen (speedwell, elatine), lupin and the juice of ivy were used for breast cancers. From the fauna, hog's grease and woman's milk were used, and well tested was the method of applying a young animal, such as a kitten or a puppy, cut in two halves, on the diseased breast. When the animal lost its natural temperature, it was replaced with a new one.[30] Many of these medications were in use in the eighteenth century as well.

Plaisters and poultices were used throughout the long century to treat the tumour from the outside. Applying pressure on the tumour with linen compresses was frequently proposed. One plaister intended to ease a 'Canker' was made with two spoonfuls of alum and honey, mixed with half a spoonful of oatmeal. Sir Kenelm Digby proposed treating breast cancer with a cataplasm made of 'an old mellow Pippin', a late sweet apple, filled with hog's grease and roasted. This was tried by Mr Bressieurs on Mrs Brent's cancerous breast, and proved good in softening the tumour.[31]

Old remedies had proved more or less ineffectual in curing cancer, and much hope was therefore placed in innovations. New World novelties were quickly welcomed as cancer medicines. In England Anthony Chute was among the first to propose tobacco as an excellent remedy because of its hot nature, and in the seventeenth century more hope was put into its effects.[32] Other 'exotic' remedies were tested as well. Guaiacum was an ingredient long used in many cancer recipes,[33] and among the fashionable seventeenth-century miracle drugs was mummy. Robert Fludd, for example, proposed mummy as an excellent cure for cancer as well as many other serious illnesses and conditions, such as 'superfluity and suppression of Menstrues in women, as also sterility in them'. It was in its nature to draw all illness out.[34] At the end of the eighteenth century favourable reports were heard about the efficacy of the Guatemalan green lizard. To receive benefit from this remedy, the patient had to swallow two or three green lizards daily. Even though the heads and tails were removed, patients found this remedy disagreeable. Nisbet wondered whether this problem could be remedied by making pills out of the lizards.[35]

In stark contrast to these expensive foreign novelties, there was still space in the Pharmacopoeia for some plain and often literally home-grown substances. At one point in the eighteenth century, carrot poultice came to be highly recommended as a treatment of ulcerated breast cancer. Grated carrot was mixed with water until it was brought to the consistency of a poultice and was applied to the ulcer in the morning and the evening. Its great advantages were undoubtedly its cheapness and ease of manufacture, but it proved to have commendable medical qualities as well: 'It generally cleans the sore, eases the pain, and takes away the disagreeable smell, which are objects of no small importance in such a dreadful disorder.'[36] Many authors recommended carrot poultice specifically because it kept the horrible stench of ulcerated cancer at bay.[37] Obviously, carrot was not expected to cure cancer, but merely to alleviate its disagreeable effects – a great quality in any substance, whether plain and familiar or foreign and exotic.

There may be nothing in carrot to suggest a revolution. However, a revolution[38] did take place from the second half of the seventeenth century onwards, both in the contents of the medicine cabinet of early modern breast cancer and in the repertoire of the breast cancer surgeon. Long before the carrot poultice was in vogue, the Paracelsians, the Helmontians, the chemists or iatrochemists had revolutionized medical thinking by renouncing Galenism: they believed that 'the best way to know the body and to understand its functioning was by means of chemistry'.[39] In Britain the influential Helmontian circle, followers of Jean Baptiste van Helmont (1579–1644), although not in support of all Paracelsus's ideas,[40] was, like the Paracelsians, driven by a revolution against Galenic medicine.[41] According to the Helmontians, cancers were caused by acrid lympha or by corroding salts.[42] There was an increasing interest in chemical medicine, all kinds of new experiments were carried out, and in effect Helmontian chemical medicine soon had an extensive cancer pharmacopoeia which increasingly turned away from the Galenic one.[43] The chemists' theory of healing was based on achieving a balance between salt, sulphur and mercury; this entailed a gradual change in the basic principles of medication in everyday practice. Where humoral theory stressed the importance of healing herbs and plants, chemical medicine put greater emphasis on metals and minerals.[44] In practical terms, chemists introduced more lethal substances into the pharmacopoeia, and it can be argued that this in part explains the professionalization of medicine: medicines were poisons, and miscalculations in the administration of medicines could easily be deadly. An intimate knowledge of these substances was needed if they were to be used safely. Their safety, it must be noted, was always considered relative. People's reactions to poisons were considered unique to the individual, which further added to the difficulties and problems surrounding their use, effectively keeping them away from the layman's reach.

Chemists introduced potent substances such as lead and mercury into the treatment of cancer, the great masters showing the way. Paracelsus had boasted of healing a woman of a cancer from which she had suffered for thirty years with 'Essentia Mercurialis, with the water of Plantaine',[45] and Van Helmont was known for his mastery in employing mercury.[46] From the seventeenth century onwards, a strenuous effort is recognizable to find one specific cure for cancer. For Galenists these cures often were compounds, for chemists simples, although such a division was more theoretical than practical. For example, Timothie

Bright and Nicholas Culpeper, leaning on the new learning, did not entirely reject the Galenic advice of combatting cancer with 'Nightshadewater, Snails boyled, and Frogs in Oyl, and with ashes of Frogs made into an Oyntment, or Medicines of Lead', since these remedies were known to alleviate pain and would not aggravate the tumour into growth.[47] Nightshade, frogs and toads were at times tested against cancer: it was even reported that a woman in Hungerford had been cured of her ulcerated breast cancer by using live toads to suck out her 'cancer poison'. Usually, however, these tests led to the simple conclusion that the substance was of no use against cancer.[48]

This search for a cure for cancer can be read as one aspect (both direct and indirect) of the new empiricism,[49] and in the case of cancer as well, the point where the most rapid changes began to take place can be (loosely) placed in the mid-seventeenth century.[50] The latter half of the seventeenth century saw many causes of wonderment in medicine and anatomy, probably the most famous of them of course being William Harvey's theory of the circulation of blood.[51] A curiosity, but worth mentioning is that when Harvey's followers experimented with blood transfusion they hoped that transfusions might also help cure cancer.[52]

As noted, the long eighteenth century provided a wealth of innovative cancer therapies: both failed shots in the dark and considerable successes (in their terms). The search for the one method of treatment which could cure breast cancer was ardent.[53] It was also highly imaginative. Electricity was a late eighteenth-century novelty which was tested on tumours in London and Edinburgh by John Brisbane and Andrew Duncan, respectively.[54] These experiments on the virtues of electricity were probably initiated by a case discussed in contemporary journals: John Leake reported the case of a gentlewoman who had been cured of a scirrhus by 'a stroke', which she had received while 'she was standing at a Window observing a heavy Thunder shower: It set fire to the thatch of the house, at the same time, forced the chimney-piece from the wall, and raised the carpet from the floor.'[55] This particular medical curiosity prompted an alertness to the possible uses of electricity in medicine, and there were reports of similar effects elsewhere. John Leake also mentioned that electricity had dispersed 'knots and Ganglions' in 'Upsal' (I take this to be Uppsala in Sweden).[56]

In Edinburgh, Andrew Duncan optimistically proposed that the aim in curing cancers should not only be to cure the disease itself but also to restore the 'parts morbidly affected to a sound state'. This ambitious goal was achieved, he proposed, 'a. by restoring a proper condition to the vessels; b. by restoring to them a due state of action.'[57]

In achieving this goal, forces such as electricity might be helpful.[58] He tested electricity on a willing patient, a sixty-two-year-old woman who could not think of having her breast cut off: 'I found her totally adverse to all thoughts of it', he reports.[59] Even though he clearly believed in experimenting with all kinds of methods, he was still a firm believer in the force of the knife in curing cancer; he concludes his book on cancer with the assertion that an operation as early as possible was the only means to try for a cure of cancer. There was no other way.[60]

While Duncan investigated the virtues of electricity, John Ewart experimented with the use of carbonic acid on ulcerated cancers of the breast. He reported on his findings in 1794, announcing one instance where the patient had been cured and another case in which the treatment had been helpful, even though this case was 'the most desperate and deplorable'. He noted that carbonic acid treatment was in no way painful and nor did it carry any risk to the patient.[61] Again we see the importance of finding a cure which the patient could easily accept, and which allowed treatment without tremendous discomfort and pain. The first of his patients was Susan Alford, a fifty-eight-year-old cook admitted to the Bath City Infirmary and Dispensary as an outpatient in June 1794. Her 'naturally large' left breast was affected with an ulcer nearly five-inches long and two-inches deep, which ran profusely. Ewart noted that the patient was in the habit of pressing the breast many times a day, and each time obtained 'from a table-spoonful to two-thirds of a small tea-cupful of very fetid matter' from the breast. He considered the patient's state pitiable.[62] Interestingly, the doctor's emotional response to his patient's state functions as part of the diagnosis and of the description of the patient's condition. It was perfectly acceptable and customary for the doctor to feel for the patient, and to write such feelings down. Empathy was a not insignificant characteristic of the medical practitioner.

Susan Alford was troubled not only with this horrible ulcer, but also by 'irregular knobs' in her breast. Her case was therefore deemed hopeless and beyond cure, which was why Ewart decided she could be treated with carbonic acid. His previous experiments with it had not been very encouraging, but had suggested there might be some advantages in the method. Testing the method on a patient with no alternative treatments available and who had only death to expect carried no significant risk to her health – or to his reputation. In other words, neither Alford nor Ewart had anything to lose.[63]

Much was actually gained, since Ewart concluded that his patient improved. Inwardly she was also given arsenic but it was attested that the carbonic acid air had made her better before any arsenic was administered. A further proof of her improvement with Ewart's method was her ecstatic response: 'the patient's expressions of relief were not cold or ambiguous, but approaching to rapture'. After a month of treatment, Ewart judged her a different woman: 'The patient had recovered her appetite, her strength, and her sleep, and was in every respect a renovated being.' By September her ulcer was healed.[64]

While electricity and carbonic acid air can be said to have been mere curiosities in the history of breast cancer therapies, it is probably safe to argue that from the late seventeenth century onwards the greatest promise (discounting surgical methods) was seen in mercury and hemlock. The popularity of these two substances had different profiles. Mercury, following the Paracelsian incursion in medicine, was seen as the universal medicine and therefore as a promising cure for cancer as well, and it maintained its importance in the following century. In contrast, hemlock, *cicuta*, was a simple, which was immensely fashionable for a short period but which, I would argue, caused the most heated debate of all among medical practitioners. First, however, a brief look at the nature of mercury as a cancer treatment is needed.

Mercury had gained enormous popularity as a universal medicine in a short time, and was soon used in the cure of cancer as well. So popular was mercury that the medical marketplace soon saw such medicines as 'Doctor Sermons most Famous and Safe Cathartique & Diuretique Pills', which were advertised as serving to expel the 'poisonous Humours' caused by mercurial remedies.[65] Notorious as a cure for syphilis, mercury was considered efficacious in cancer because of its drying quality: it would, it was hoped, shrink tumours. This is why so many women with breast cancers were salivated with mercury. As always, support for the virtues of mercury was not unanimous; in the late eighteenth century, Burrows, for example, was sceptical about its virtues.[66] But positive voices were far more frequent. Thomas Marryat and Robert White both recommended mercury for expelling early cancers, and considered the knife and mercury as the two main options for the patient.[67] Mercury was also used in palliative care. In his *Domestic Medicine* William Buchan endorsed mercurial pills and mercurial ointment as part of a regimen for keeping cancer symptoms at bay.[68] Joseph Higgs, a Birmingham surgeon, advertised having cured numerous cancer patients with mercury. For example, Mrs Baker, a gentlewoman, had earlier been pronounced by specialists to be incurable, but Higgs's treatment cured her, and a similarly happy ending was brought about for Mrs Harris from Moor Street in Birmingham.[69]

While mercury seems to have been quietly in wide use against cancer, hemlock (most often used in the form of *cicuta vulgaris*) caused an exceptionally lively exchange of ideas and theoretical debate in the latter part of the eighteenth century. Great hopes were placed in its virtues. The debate and experimentation on hemlock in Britain was initiated by the translation of Anton Störck's [Stork] *An Essay in Hemlock*, which focused specifically on curing cancer. The book, published in English in Aberdeen in 1762, claimed that Störck had cured several cancer patients using hemlock.[70] Defending his controversial discovery, he claimed that the use of the plant for medical purposes was not his own invention but had been practised by the ancients; he further noted that its usefulness had been tainted by its extremely poisonous nature. By first testing it on 'a little dog that was hungry' and later on himself, he realized that hemlock was not lethal if used in suitable doses. Careful dosages were indeed needed; when he took too much of it, he explained, his tongue swelled up, and he temporarily lost the power of speech.[71]

Störck's news about the usefulness of hemlock was immediately eagerly received in Britain, and it was tested locally. After just a few years, however, the news spread that *cicuta* was useless or of only limited use às a palliative remedy, and that the British plant was different and less effective than German hemlock.[72] Richard Guy presented twenty cancer cases (of which fourteen were cancers in the breast and one was uncertain but probably in the breast) in which hemlock had been used by other doctors before the patients saw Guy: hemlock brought the patients nothing but drowsiness, nausea, fainting spells, blindness – one patient was paralysed even – and all this for nothing, Guy attested, since their tumours continued to grow.[73] While the debate continued, hemlock was easily assigned the blame if a patient's situation grew worse. In the middle of the debate in London, the wife of the Russian ambassador Alexei Semionovich Musin-Pushkin (1744–1817, ambassador to London from 1769 to 78) was to the horror of some of the medical profession given hemlock for a scirrhous tumour in her breast. When her tumour turned cancerous, this specific treatment was quickly believed to be the cause:

> Two weeks more had hardly elapsed, when Dr. N—r, paying me a visit, told me, that the lady, in consequence of her *hemlock-pills*, and *hemlock-fumigations to the breast*, was brought to the last extremity; but that, bad as she was, if I would wait on her, he did not doubt but she would be happy to put herself once more under my care. Prompted by respect for a worthy family, and by a humanity, which, I hope, will never forsake me, I accordingly waited on the Ambassador; but such was the condition of the lady, when I called, that I could not see her. I had, nevertheless, a long conference with his Excellency; nor could I take my leave of him, without solemnly declaring, that the methods taken with his lady would terminate in her death. She had fallen into hands, however, from which it was not easy to extricate her.[74]

The lady was then removed to Russia (this removal was probably connected with the ending of her husband's posting to London in 1778). The writer mentions that her cancerous breast was cut off in Russia, and that she perished: 'Thus closed a tragedy', he laments, 'of which the unhappy heroine, still lamented by all who had the honour of her acquaintance, was allowed to be one of the most amiable and most accomplished women who ever visited a British court.'[75]

It is important to remember that although hemlock was often considered dangerous and controversial, it was also recommended for cancer especially if there was little hope left for the patient. Its use, however, needed to be based on common sense and professional judgement. As its side-effects were known, it was agreed that some reservations in its use were necessary: 'Some tender habits will not bear it, as it affects the head; but its usefulness will fully compensate some slight inconveniencies. Begin with smaller doses in young people.'[76]

Hemlock was typically taken in the form of pills and extract, but Justamond, the surgeon of Westminster Hospital, also used it as a bath. It was used in great quantities; he mentions 30 pounds of hemlock used in one bath. To be effective the solution had to be strong, thus causing high fever, convulsions and great pain.[77] Medicated baths were fashionable for a time; they were considered potentially very effective, since the patient was completely immersed in the substance which was believed to treat her cancer. Bath therapy could be taken at home as well if one could afford a bathtub.[78]

Treating Pain

Before discussing the surgical treatments of cancer, let us take a look at the treatment of pain, an ever-present fact of life in early modern Europe. In her admirable analysis, Barbara Duden reminds us about the inevitability of early modern pain:

> Whether pain was seen as Hippocratic disharmony, as a Platonic deficiency in the mode of existence, as a Manichaean mistake of the demiurge, or as a result of the Christian fall from grace, these perceptions were based on the notion that pain expressed the broken state of nature. Pain could thus be endured or overcome, at best it could be alleviated, calmed, soothed, but fighting it would have been meaningless. A sufferer could defy pain, try to deny it, submit to it, but he could not escape it.[79]

Indeed there was great need to keep the pains of illness at bay, to make pain as unnoticeable as possible. While pain could not be conquered, weapons against it were available, and a great deal of effort went into relieving pain, whether it was toothache, headache or cancer pain. With time, more attention was also paid to the possibilities of sedation during surgery and other intense pain.[80] Of more immediate relevance, however, was relieving pain. Robert Mustow, in his commonplace book (1663–5), listed a number of efficient medications. First, he recommended trying anodynes or 'paregoricall' medications, which we would call painkillers. These were either simple anodynes (made of a single substance), such as the roots of althea, mallow, lilies; leaves of the same; seeds of hemp, marshmallow and fenugreek; flowers of lilies, chamomile, and 'melilott'; or compounds (mixtures of several substances), such as oils of sweet almonds or lilies.[81] Thus a single seventeenth-century surgical commonplace book offered quite an arsenal of plants to use against pain. These plants had traditionally been used for pain medication, for instance in cataplasms (poultices) to alleviate the pain caused by tumours, or in the form of a liniment, as suggested by Banister in his famous *An Antidotarie chyrurgicall*, to 'delay paine in malignant cancerous ulcers'.[82] Two hundred years later, Bryan Cornwell recommended treating a very painful ulcerated cancer with bleeding, purging, a lean cooling diet and inward anodynes. Additionally, 'destroying the sensibility of the parts by preparations of lead' would be useful.[83] This 'destroying the sensibility' inevitably leads to the question of the pains arising from surgical operations.

Surgical anaesthesia was not practised before the nineteenth century,[84] and it is futile to try to completely separate painkilling from sedation concerning earlier times. While it was being tested here and there during the latter eighteenth century, anaesthesia against pain was not commonly pursued. According to Latta, there were two options for rendering 'the operation more tolerable': the first consisted of substances such as opium, the other, he thought, was

> compressing the nerve which goes to the part to be operated upon, so that it cannot feel pain so acutely as it would otherwise do. Opium would be perfectly [*sic*] answer the first intention, were not its effects upon the system to be dreaded. Large doses of this medicine are very apt to bring on sickness and vomiting, which, after some operations, are much to be dreaded; and therefore its use is laid aside by the most judicious practitioners. A machine for compressing the nerves was invented by Mr James Moore of London ... It is designed to compress the nerves so completely, that the parts below it may be altogether insensible, and thus the operation be performed absolutely without pain to the patient. A difficulty, however, occurs here. To produce this perfect insensibility, the nerves must be compressed at least an hour; and, as they always lie near the large veins, there is danger of taking in some of the latter along with them; and such a long continued compression on a vein would be in danger of causing it burst. To remedy this, Mr Moore proposes to open a vein; but, unless in robust patients, this could not be done; so that, until the machine can be brought to such perfection that we can certainly compress the nerves without the veins, we cannot expect from it those advantages which it otherwise promises.[85]

We will return below to the effects of opium, which Latta also notes. Very interesting is also the report on James Moore's nerve compression machine. This was a serious attempt to produce an unfailing method to bring patients freedom from pain – without the disadvantages and dangers of putting them to sleep, which we will revisit shortly.

For us, the premodern reluctance to anaesthetize patients is perhaps difficult to understand. Resistance against using medications that would induce sleep in operations was formidable – but logically founded. Mustow noted that only if anodynes failed should one resort to 'Narcotic Medicamentes'.[86] This reluctance to put a patient to sleep even during the most agonizing operation was based on at least four well-founded reasons: First, it was important for the patient to remain conscious, so that, in case death ensued (and following the ideal of a 'good death'), one died conscious and in a state of holy repentance. This theological explanation probably carried far into the eighteenth century, if not further, and was probably very important to patients. Another explanation comes from the field of medicine itself: narcotic medications were dangerous, in fact often lethal. Thirdly, the surgeon needed the patient conscious in order to follow her state.[87] And finally, many writers considered pain useful, even necessary, in the process of healing. Indeed it was argued that sedatives brought about less successful outcomes than surgeries without sedatives.[88] The line between sleep and death was arguably thin, and caution was needed. Mustow's commonplace book notes in a section titled 'A Phisical Dictionarie' that 'Narcoticks' are 'stupifying medicines: which dull the sence of ye feeling & cause deepe sleepe'.[89] Without doubt, deep sleep was dangerously death-like.

So feared was a state of deep sleep that it is exceptional to find any accounts of mastectomies in which it was considered advantageous. If fainting can be counted as such a state, one exception can be found in James Hill's report on Miss J— M—, in which he notes that 'At the first touch of the instrument, she fortunately fainted, and did not fully recover till the operation was finished, and the dressings applied'. Even though Hill mentions that 'she fortunately fainted', after a few lines he nevertheless writes that her fainting in fact brought dangers with it since it increased the hemorrhage: 'Her fainting had prevented the springing of the arteries, and put it out of our power to tie them, or to apply pledgets to each. This accident gave me much uneasiness.' Hill's contradictory views, the fainting being on the one hand fortunate for the patient, on the other giving him 'much uneasiness', can be understood through his dual role. Her fainting brought about a situation which for him as a surgeon was 'an accident' and professionally difficult; as a human being, however, he felt it was fortunate for her since she felt little or nothing of the operation.[90]

The 'Narcotic Medicamentes' included very strong substances, ones that had been in use since times beyond memory: mandrake, henbane, hemlock, waterlily and poppy;[91] of the chemical medicine cabinet, he recommended, for example Sydenham's 'Laudanum opiate'.[92] Roy Porter argues that the most popular premodern painkiller was alcohol,[93] but while alcohol was indeed in very widespread use, it was opium that seems to have dominated the medical debate. Furthermore, it would be safe to argue that in the eighteenth century opium replaced alcohol, especially in the treatment of elite patients.[94] As Roselyne Rey notes, in the eighteenth century resorting to opium was the norm – in contrast to the previous century, when there was some disagreement about its virtues, and when especially influential French surgeons opposed its use.[95]

In 1700, John Jones explicated in *The Mysteries of Opium* its many uses: it could be used to 'to cause Sleep, take away Pain, &c.',[96] Opium was prescribed for breast cancer patients not only for numbing the pain but also as a medication to resolve the tumour, since one of opium's good qualities was understood to be its powerful ability to soften hardness. Opium was used both internally and externally, but the patient about to undergo amputation would most commonly receive it in the form of a cordial. To be effective, the cordial had to be taken in advance; it took half an hour for liquid opium to take effect, and perhaps up to an hour and a half for solid opium to do so.[97]

In the late eighteenth century, Henry Fearon warned against the use of these stimulating cordials before operations, because they increased bleeding and hence added to the dangers of the operation. He noted that well-meaning friends and relatives had to be kept an eye on: he hinted it was not unusual for the patient to receive such a cordial before an operation unbeknownst to the surgeon. The patient had to be guarded against such folly, he thought: even though the friends – or, as he put it, 'the tender sympathizing nurse' – meant well in wanting to help the patient bear the operation better, they actually added to the latter's sufferings because the cordials weakened the patient.[98]

George Young was more positive about the virtues of opium. In his *Treatise on Opium* he wrote that fear added to the dangers of an amputation, at its worst causing convulsions during the operation. To avoid this, opium given two or three hours prior to an operation would 'give courage and steddiness [*sic*] both of body and mind'. It would not, he added, 'abate the pain of the operation, as the patient expected; but it makes him better able to bear it'.[99] Young at first thought that opium was excellent in cases of cancers in the breast: 'The great temporary relief procured by opium, at a time when nothing else did any service, made me than fix it as a rule, that opium, and nothing else, was of service in a cancerated breast; and the immediate good effects of it easily convinced others, that the observation was right'.[100]

But, as noted, we should not imagine that opium removed the sense of pain. Fanny Burney was fully awake and sensible during her mastectomy operation, and an eighteenth-century amputee has described the removal of a limb:

> During the operation, in spite of the pain it occasioned, my senses were preternaturally acute, as I have been told they generally are in patients under such circumstances ... I still recall with unwelcome vividness the spreading out of the instruments, the twisting of the tourniquet, the first incision, the fingering of the sawed bone, the sponge pressed, on the flap, the tying of the blood-vessels, the stitching of the skin, and the bloody dismembered limb lying on the floor.[101]

Even though it did not remove acute sensations of pain of surgery, opium was a substance that released the long-lasting agonies of cancer. It was also seen as a friend to the dying. There is plentiful evidence that cancer patients were given opium during their illness in order to relieve their pain. John Hunter mentions this explicitly in the case of Mrs Farhill: 'She also took Opium occasionally to relieve her of the Pain'.[102] Buchan notes in his *Domestic Medicine* that opium was 'a kind of solace', the one medicine to which one could resort when everything else failed. Opium 'will not indeed cure the disease', he wrote, 'but it will ease the patient's agony, and render life more tolerable while it continues'.[103] All in all, it can be concluded that opium brought some but not complete release from extreme pain, helped in the palliative treatment of dying patients, and was quite often used in surgery, especially in the eighteenth century. That said, it is now time for us to turn our gaze to the surgical treatment of cancer in the breast.

'The Dreadful Necessity of having Recourse to the Knife':[104]
Surgical Operations

Early modern surgery was frightening, extremely dangerous, and at times considered a 'dreadful necessity'. Surgeons had two methods available in treating cancer: cautery and surgery. Cautery basically meant burning, and was performed with hot irons; burning with medications was often called caustic remedy as well. Surgery was carried out with knives, scalpels and other such instruments. In the treatment of cancer, both methods were in use in the removal of tumours and whole breasts. There was no unanimity as to the worth, efficacy or results of the two approaches. In general, cautery was usually deemed less certain in its effectiveness against cancer, even in cases where the whole breast was removed by cautery, and many were suspicious of caustic methods. However, one must bear in mind that cautery with burning irons was used in knife surgery as well. Since cautery was a long drawn-out process – it could take months to remove a cancerous breast with corrosives such as arsenic – many surgeons considered it far more painful than removal of the breast by the knife.[105]

Early modern surgery is often portrayed as a field in which there was little improvement, but a few important innovations in surgical techniques did take place from the late seventeenth century onwards. There was great interest in improving surgical techniques, and new ideas were constantly proposed.[106] While no definite figures are available, I feel confident in suggesting that surgical operations for breast cancers became more common during the period. This development provided more operative patients as subjects for surgical research, while improved techniques in turn meant greater willingness to undergo an operation. Again, empathy towards patients was a strong force in the development of less painful surgical methods: better techniques were needed to lessen what was rightly considered the unimaginable pain of the operations. Some of the innovations could be described as revolutions. New instruments were designed to enable faster cutting and to save the patient from excess suffering. In the following I discuss the techniques involved in the surgical treatment of cancers in the breast, and cast light on the many aspects of the perennial debate and argument as to whether the patient actually benefited from surgery – and, it followed, whether in general it was worth using the knife.

To understand the scope of the ongoing discussion and the great variety of methods available in the attempt to cure cancer, let us take a look at cautery. In the early eighteenth century, the surgeon William Beckett rejected all treatment of cancer both by the knife and by cautery (nor did he accept salivation with mercury), and suggested that the illness could only be cured by a special dissolvent which consumed the cancer and eliminated it in three weeks.[107] While he did not see his dissolvent as a form of cautery, such dissolvents were nevertheless included among caustic methods by many of his colleagues, and were strictly rejected by many of them. One such example is Lorenz Heister, who warned against the use of any repelling or astringent remedies against cancer. These, he claimed, would increase the disease 'wonderfully', adding that 'one Month will produce more Increase of Pain and Tumour, than a Year without any medicinal Applications' – and would produce an ulcer.[108] Since ulcers were generally considered incurable, this in fact meant that medicating the cancer shortened the patient's life; a medicating surgeon, it was implied, thus acted as an angel of death.

In the latter part of the eighteenth century, William Rowley supported treating cancers with medications, but not with caustic ones. He too considered all cautery suspicious, suitable only for quacks. Cautery, he argued, whether in the form of burning irons or of caustic substances, was agonizing for patients, and made their lives miserable. Rowley's attitude towards quacks was negative throughout: 'considerable mischief is done both by the knife and caustic. This last, is the remedy of the secret curers, who artfully call every disease of the breast a cancer; imposing a method of cure on their patients, too cruel for any surgeon to practice.'[109] Rowley's suspicion reflects the perennial discussion as to who was to be allowed to treat ill people and who was not. Even though cautery was an everyday part of surgery, the problem was that quacks were notorious for the use of caustic substances; and quacks of course were and had been enemies to surgeons and physicians alike. In the battle over the foundation of medical authority, the methods of the quacks had already been exposed and deemed dubious in the sixteenth century as well as later. But William Rowley, who was himself a surgeon, should be seen as an exceptionally critical practitioner. If he was harsh with his judgements, he similarly seems to have thought little of his colleagues' skills in healing breast cancer patients. He bluntly accuses surgeons of actually killing their patients:

> I was recommended by Her Grace the Dutchess of — [Portland], to Mrs. P—, who had a cancerous complaint in her breast. She had been for near two years under the care of a surgeon, who asserted, with confidence, that she would certainly be cured. She applied caustics to some hardened tumours under the arm, as likewise to the breast; and it was reported, that he had given some preparations of arsenic; this last circumstance, however, can scarce be credited, we should hope it not true. The ulcer where the caustics had been applied was at least an inch and half deep, and four or five inches long, discharging a most offensive matter. She was in exquisite tortures day and night. At first sight of the case, I pronounced it incurable, to the noble friends of the patient; and all that could be attempted, was a mitigation of the symptoms. The ulcerated parts were dressed with the ung. saturninum with camphor. The pulvis mineralis was given in small doses, and considerable ease was procured. The putridity of the discharge, however, and the other miserable circumstances of the case, brought on hectical symptoms; a difficulty of breathing every day increased, and the patient died, most probably a victim of the pretended knowledge and cruel practices of her surgeon.[110]

Rowley accused the surgeon not only of lack of skill but of using arsenic as a caustic medicine. As Rowley was not a supporter of those who believed cancer was caused by acidity, he did not consider arsenic a worthy alkaline medicine to use against the disease.[111] There were deep disagreements as to the nature of some of the caustic substances used in professional medicine; one of the most widely debated was without doubt arsenic. While Rowley and others attacked it fiercely, its use in breast cancer was not unusual and had a long history – it is not exceptional to find arsenic mentioned in sixteenth-century medical treatises. In the eighteenth century, arsenic was much used and yet under heavy suspicion by many.[112] Justamond for example opposed the use of arsenic as a simple because it was too painful: the pain caused by the substance continued too long after it was applied to the tumour. He nevertheless found arsenic in compound medicines useful in advanced cases, and proposed that a combination of opium and arsenic used in cautery eased the pain; ultimately he decided that an arsenic mixture was the most effective external application available. He also tested arsenic as an internal medicine.[113]

To return to Rowley, it is interesting that he accused the surgeon of the well-connected patient's death; he did not see the devastating disease as the culprit, even though the cancer had spread widely. It is plain that Rowley was making politics by his rash statement. In treating cancer patients, he asserted, the wise doctor – like himself – would most often leave the disease untreated. In the case of a disease like cancer, it was the role of the doctor in most cases to be a 'true friend' and advise the patient to submit to the course of nature.[114] Patience would actually add years to a patient's life, he felt. The other kind of surgeon, Rowley pointed out, especially the young, the inexperienced, and those who were 'devoid of feeling' would 'rashly' seize a knife and operate.[115]

Mastectomies

What caused most horror and 'melancholy instances', to quote Rowley, in women with tumours in their breasts, however, were not caustic substances but the thought of surgery. Of all surgical procedures, mastectomy – complete removal of the breast – was among the most feared. Both medical practitioners and patients considered mastectomy especially cruel. Some patients, however, were eligible for extirpation, an operation to remove a smallish tumour from the breast which saved the rest of the breast. An extirpation was possible if the patient was youngish and otherwise healthy, and had a relatively small and loose tumour. It must be noted that not all practitioners considered extirpation an option at all; they felt that not removing all of the breast tissue would leave cancerous matter in the breast and thus cause certain death.[116] From the patient's perspective, however, extirpation must have been much easier to consent to.

The surgeon William Norford, for example, had a patient who was extremely reluctant to have her very diseased breast removed, but who expressed no great distaste against having her tumour itself extirpated. Norford noted that her reluctance to undergo a mastectomy was reflected in the very 'dejected' and melancholy position he found her sitting in when he saw her. The patient's overall appearance changed when she learned her breast could be saved.[117] Clearly, saving her breast was important for her – it was the thought of mastectomy that had made her miserable, not the thought of surgery in general.

The suffering of patients was understood by laymen and medical practitioners alike. In fact, it was difficult for practitioners to distance themselves from the experiences of their patients. As Linda Payne has shown, learning medical dispassion was far from easy, and it was especially gruelling for many practitioners to carry out such surgical operations as mastectomies on living patients.[118] One could not distance oneself too much, however, since the proper ethics of a surgeon included a degree of empathy and understanding for the patient and her suffering. Appositely in this context, Pierre Dionis noted with some regret that the breasts, the ornaments of the fair sex, were 'frequently oblig'd to undergo very cruel Operations'.[119] Ethically, it was also paramount for the physician to carefully consider the patient's chances of surviving an operation, both physically and mentally. One aspect of this consideration was the well-known fact that the benefits of surgery were always uncertain: no method of treatment could promise a cancer patient a cure.

This uncertainty played a part in the debate over the merits of the knife in cases of cancers of the breast, which continued during the whole of the period covered here. The discussion reflects the extent of knowledge of cancers, and suggests the various directions which practitioners of medicine were willing to take in their ongoing search for a cure. Approaching the debate in chronological terms, we can attempt to evaluate the importance of surgery in the different centuries under consideration. We have to begin with tradition, and with the sixteenth century, when it was well known that Hippocrates and Galen had been sceptical about the benefits of surgery. Of the great and 'ancient' authorities, Avicenna (980–1037) was more inclined to favour an operation as a possible treatment. It was reported that Avicenna 'woulde haue it [the cancer tumour] taken away by incision, if so be it be not dangerous to the part where it is.'[120] This accurately sums up the general sixteenth-century idea that an operation in itself was worth consideration if the tumour was small enough and was in a suitable place, especially not very deep in the breast. Where most surgeons would probably have considered removing a small tumour from the top of the breast, there were well-founded reasons for serious reservations against treating ulcerous cancers; these were seen as an especially grave problem; they were 'vile' and resisted all treatment.[121]

It is difficult if not impossible to determine whether the seventeenth century saw a greater inclination towards surgery. Many surgeons were still very cautious about treating cancers in general, and were not eager to perform with the knife.[122] Popular medicine, including advice books such as *The Compleat Doctoress* (1656), continued to uphold the position that advanced or ulcerated cases should receive only palliative treatment.[123]

However, there were also those who more possibilities and benefits to surgery than their abovementioned colleagues, particularly among French medical practitioners. Barthélemy Saviard rejected the cautious attitude of Hippocrates and Celsius; he emphasized the need to consider each and every case individually, rather than systematically opposing an operation in cases which, even though advanced, promised positive results.[124] Even more optimistic voices were heard. Paul Barbette, who practised in Amsterdam, seems to have considered surgery the best answer to most cancers, especially those not ulcerated, but care had to be taken not to leave any cancer behind in the wound.[125] At the turn of the eighteenth century, John Moyle quite radically argued in his *The Experienced Chirurgion* that cancer was only curable by the knife.[126]

We should not think of the eighteenth century as a triumphal century of the scalpel. There were many surgeons who believed cancer was incurable by the knife. Indeed, one of the most prolific surgeon-writers, William Rowley, constantly exhorted his colleagues to keep their knives at bay, and not to operate on cancers except under very special circumstances. According to him, the knife was simply futile.[127] Regardless of this continuous doubt, the eighteenth century saw a substantial rise in interest in breast cancer. The French surgeons were publishing at an accelerating speed, but their English and Scottish colleagues soon caught up with them.

Rejecting pessimism, many eighteenth-century surgeons now saw themselves as seeking a cure. It was Dale Ingram who expressed their quest with perhaps the greatest eloquence:

> Accordingly the Mathematician labours for the Discovery of the Longitude and the Quadrature of the Circle, and the Physician is impatient to know wherein the genuine and latent Principle of Life consists. In this respect the Surgeon has the manifest Advantage of the other two; since he aims at no particular Point, farther than the Cure of his patient, which in many Cases may be obtained by an accurate Knowledge of the Parts he operates upon, and a sufficient Degree of Consideration and Experience. As this is the Case, we may justly be surprized, that Surgery has made no greater Advances than to be looked upon as something not only precarious and uncertain, but even as a Kind of Jest contrived to drain the Pockets and amputate the Limbs of Mankind.[128]

Ingram concludes by noting that surgeons were often the object of ridicule and mockery, which they found incomprehensible.

When we look at the eighteenth-century debate on breast cancer, it is evident that changes – sometimes fundamental – were taking place both in surgical technique and in the areas of ethics and attitudes.

Encouragement to use the knife more often came from French surgeons as well. Pierre Dionis can be seen as a representative of the change that took place in attitudes towards operating on more difficult and more advanced cancers. In practice, it seems, surgeons were already operating on cases that were clearly hopeless – an activity which a few decades ago would have been largely considered unethical. Attitudes, it seems, had changed in a generation. Surgeons now carried out more risky operations because of their good will towards their patients; the latter begged that their terribly diseased breasts be cut off. Even though he knew he was speaking against the ancient ideal, Dionis boldly argued the case of these desperate patients:

> But how are you to resist the Persecutions of a poor suffering Patient, which implores your Help? Are you to abandon her to the Rigour of her Distemper, which torments her Day and Night? No, a Chirurgeon must not be so cruel: He must search out Means to cure her: And if that is not in his Power, he must at least endeavour to soften the Disease, and render it more supportable.[129]

Dionis argued that the knife could ease the sufferings of patients, even of those who had little hope left. No longer was a cure the only acceptable motive for using the knife; prolonging life or diminishing the patient's pain was becoming an increasingly valid reason to operate. It is possible that earlier surgeons already operated on desperate cases, and that the debate merely made public an already common practice; but this is something we cannot really know. In any case, there was a shift in attitude: it was now possible to discuss in published texts the option of operating on patients whose lives could not be saved.

The suitable moment for an operation remained open to debate. By the latter half of the eighteenth century, four different attitudes towards the virtues of surgery can be observed. Some writers considered only early and small unattached cancers to be operable;[130] others thought that surgery was the best treatment in advanced cases;[131] the third group could consider these radical operations; while finally, the fourth felt there was nothing one could actually do to save a cancer patient.

Urgency became the keyword. As already mentioned, many writers thought that an operation had to be carried out as soon as possible in order to prevent the cancer virus from spreading.[132] This resonates with present-day medical practices and women's self-help campaigns, which put the patient on the frontline: women have a duty to check their breasts regularly because 'early detection' is the key to treating cancer. Back in the eighteenth century, Andrew Duncan agreed with Hill, who had written that 'were it my fate to be affected with cancer, I would not delay operation a single hour'.[133] Benjamin Bell insisted on amputating every small ulcer in the breast immediately; cancers, he noted, were of local origin, and any ulcer in the breast might make the cancer to absorb elsewhere in the breast. The breast was a dangerous locus: a cancer located there was more apt to be absorbed widely everywhere in the body than one located anywhere else. This, he said pointedly, should be the very cause of immediate amputation of the breast. He was quite adamant, in fact, that 'in every instance where the parts affected can be safely separated from the sound, as nothing but their removal can afford any chance of safety, I must again say, that we should not hesitate to advise the operation'.[134]

The point of this urgency, as Brookes insisted, was to catch the monster before it could 'be exasperated and strike inwards, generate others, and increase those already formed'.[135] In practice, this meant that the tumour had to be cut off before it turned cancerous. As theory and actual patient care often remained widely separated, in practice this seems to have been rarely the case. Buchan describes the delays which normally took place: 'Few people will submit to the extirpation till death stares them in the face; whereas, if it were done early, the patient would be in no danger of losing his life by the operation, and it would generally prove a radical cure.'[136]

Buchan himself left open the alternative of waiting, noting that if the tumour enlargened and hardened, one should operate.[137] The Edinburgh Practice (1800) similarly proposed a rapid approach; since in advanced cases the prognosis was extremely bad, one should take action at a point where the tumour had not yet turned from a schirrus into cancer.[138]

The third group of authors were those who considered operations possible even on very advanced cases. Benjamin Gooch was of the opinion that a very early operation could save the patient, but he attested that he had operated successfully on malignant cancers as well; not only that, he had with good success operated on two patients with cancers already ulcerated or metastasized (to use a present-day term) to the axilla.[139] This was encouraging news for many sufferers. Decades earlier, in the first half of the eighteenth century, Samuel Sharp had likewise reported operating on patients with cancers which had spread to these lymph nodes. In cases where they could be removed without cutting the large arteries, 'they have not laid backwards and deep', he felt there was no need not to operate.[140] Henry Fearon too was radical: he argued that it was often beneficial to operate on advanced cases as well, if for no other reason than to ease the life of the patient, so that she would not be 'left a victim to the fury of this disease'.[141] White wrote that 'nothing absolutely prohibits' an operation unless it would in practice mean killing the patient.[142] This meant that only if the surgeon knew that the patient had no chance of surviving the operation itself should surgery be avoided. In all other cases the knife would bring some hope or measure of relief.

Fearon was optimistic, and considered that with early extirpation the patient had a chance to live to an old age;[143] indeed it was the duty of every practitioner to relieve the miserable, 'miseriris succurrere'.[144] For him, too, operating early on was essential; as warning examples he described two patients (mentioning he knew of other similar cases) who without an operation had died within just days, even though their cases gave no signs of being aggressive.[145]

According to the fourth group, whom we might easily refer to as 'medical pessimists', Fearon could not have been more wrong. Nisbet, for example, was strictly opposed to Hill's conclusions; he claimed that Hill had operated on schirrhi, not cancers, and had thus operated on patients who had not required an operation at all.[146] He went on to note 'that in genuine Cancer of the breast, it [surgery] has very generally failed; even the most favourable cases being only a temporary alleviation'. He based this conclusion on 'having attended particularly to all the cases of extirpation for the last thirty years in the metropolis, under the most eminent surgeons'.[147] What spoke more strongly against operating, according to Nisbet, was what was accepted as a generally acknowledged fact: that after a relapse the pains of cancer were worse than before.[148] These relapses were notoriously difficult to anticipate: if there was no relapse in the wound area, in some cases the patient was completely free of the disease while in others the cancer emerged in some other location – perhaps several years after extirpation.[149]

Nisbet, however, may provide us with indirect evidence that the pendulum was moving towards favouring surgical treatment of cancer rather than merely medical or palliative care. The first edition of his *The Clinical Guide* in 1793 listed the physician's treatments of breast cancer, but omitted surgery. The second edition, published in 1800, now noted that modern surgery was advanced compared to that of the ancients, one of the criteria being healing by the first intention (of which more later).[150] Still conservative and pessimistic in his views, Nisbet refrained from being overly excited about the new developments in surgery and about its benefits, reminding his readers that '[i]n spite, however, of these boasted advantages of treatment, the records of every hospital show the inefficacy of surgery, as well as medicine, in the cure of this form of disease'.[151] The unchanging undercurrent in all writing was that human beings were quite helpless when facing this tremendous foe, which worked in mischievous ways one could not fully understand.

This pessimism was deepest in those who thought that cancer was a disorder brought about by a general disorder of the system, i.e. not a local disease; there was therefore no hope of curing it, and the knife would not help. In these terms, Monro was quite sceptical as to the benefits of surgery, and thought that operations should only be carried out on patients who were young and fit. This was because almost in every case the cancer would return. Of his own cancer cases (which also included other forms besides breast cancer) he had seen only four people out of sixty alive and without cancer after two years.[152]

With such poor success rates, many thought surgeons too knife-happy. George Coltman for instance scoffed, citing Ovid, at surgeons who refused to see the benefits of other remedies. The problem was that

> [h]ackneyed in one common road of treatment, surgeons, whose dexterity lies in action, seldom trouble themselves with thought: if the case yield not to the usual mode of treatment, the malignancy of the disease is pronounced insuperable by the milder powers of medicines, and the beloved knife is brandished with an 'Ense recidendum, ne pars sincera trahatur'.[153]

Jean Astruc was highly pessimistic about the prognosis of cancer: whether one amputated the breast or used palliative care alone, there was no hope except to extend the life of the patient. Astruc in fact admitted he had seen cures of cancer in cases of young women whose cancer had arisen from an outward cause (such as a blow). This in his opinion was the only reasonable diagnosis justifying an operation, since only such cases offered any hope. Indeed, if the cause was inward, or if the cancer had adhered to the pectoral muscle or sides or spread to the armpit, there was no point in operating. Similarly there was no hope if the patient was menopausal, had irregular menstruation or was cacochymic (ill-humoured).[154] Astruc's view was supported in England by some, such as John Ball, who also posited that younger women whose schirrhi were caused by bruises could perhaps be saved.[155]

John Burrows proposed only palliative treatment for cancer, which perhaps reflects his profession as a physician rather than a surgeon. Thus, in treating a patient one had to pay attention to internal and external remedies, relieving pain, stopping the frequent haemorrhages, and of course keep to a proper regimen (regular sleep, diet and exercise).[156] In passing sentence against amputation, Burrows was eloquent:

> it is in vain to expect success from amputation, whilst the morbid matter remains still fixed in the juices ... the disease will break out again either in the same place, or throw itself upon some other part; the cancerous lurking humour, being, as it were, conveyed thither by a kind of metastasis or translation of the peccant matter.[157]

But whatever their method, no one considered cancer easy to cure; for everyone cancer was a tremendous foe. Opinions as to the chances offered by surgery, as we have seen, varied greatly. Some writers believed that surgery in some cases had its advantages, and that it prolonged life; according to others, it shortened life or at worst brought immediate death. Because of the elusive nature of the disease – let us bear in mind that even today breast cancer is not fully understood – this was inevitable. Since breast cancer remained a mystery, the patient had to decide among many choices: different understandings of cancer, different treatments, and different prognoses of the disease.

Surgical Techniques

Let us now take a look at what happened to those patients who chose to treat their cancers in the breast by a surgical operation, with a few words on the main principles of cancer surgery; this will be followed by a chronological overview of the techniques favoured during the period between the sixteenth and the nineteenth century. As far as the main principles of surgery are concerned, throughout the early modern period it seems to have been a commonplace for the ideal surgeon to be gentle yet thorough. It would not do to cut a small incision to the breast and then leave any diseased parts behind. Everything diseased had to be removed.[158]

According to the main principles of humoral pathology, it was considered advisable to operate on cancers only during spring and autumn. Summers were too hot, winters too cold for the body to adapt optimally to the operation: 'through the great heat of the Summer the Spirits be resolved; or by reason of the extream cold in the Winter the native heat should be choaked'.[159] This rule was relaxed when the Galenic system gave way, but in practice some of the ancient ways were continuously applied. At the end of the eighteenth century, Gooch, for example, suggested that there had perhaps been too much relaxation of these ancient maxims, and that more care was needed in preparing for surgery. When the patient was a woman, it was important to wait until her menstrual discharge was completely over, and to operate a few days later.[160] Similarly, purging the patient before the operation remained common throughout the eighteenth century.

Our survey of mastectomy techniques begins with a breast operation in 1587:

> Let the patient lye on her back, and first cut the sound part of the brest, & presently after the incision seare it, to procure a crust vpon it, which wil stay the fluxe of bloud: Not long after make incision againe to the bottome of the brest, with often searifiyng, then also seare it both cutting & searing must bee often vsed.[161]

From the very first incision, the goal of healing the wound well afterwards was to be kept in mind. It is important to note that the wound was always left open and treated with various medications, including cataplasms; the body was in a sense left to heal itself, to form scar tissue. Recovery took months, and was without doubt indescribably painful.

As mentioned earlier, the frequency of surgical operations seems to have increased in the seventeenth century. The print medium was a great force, and medicine was among the fields that gained interest among the ever-growing reading public. Surgeons could gain great fame; this was an age of famous surgeons, such as Adrian Hélvetius in Paris, who was well noted for his innovations in the treatment of cancer. He boasted that he personally had introduced breast operations in France, and had invented special pliers, 'the Helvetian forceps', to separate the tumour from the breast tissue to ease the severing of the breast.[162] This invention came to replace another seventeenth-century technique, that of using cords, because forceps was considered more humane.[163] Again, techniques and cancer treatments were developed and planned keeping the interest of the patient in mind.

The cord technique was widely used in the seventeenth century. The surgeon pierced the breast with large needles (alternatively one could use a hook or a fork) to draw threads through the breast. He would then pull the cords to separate the breast from the chest to ease cutting.[164] William Beckett describes the technique in his *Practical Surgery* (1740). His patient was a forty-year-old woman who had an aggressive tumour which eventually ulcerated. She finally consulted a surgeon, who with his colleagues proposed that the breast be cut off. She acquiesced, and the operation went as follows:

> A convenient Place being chosen, the Patient was seated on the End of a Form, a Servant being placed behind her, to confine her in that Posture, and another on the right side to sustain the sound Breast that it might receive no Damage during the Operation. Then the Operator passed a Needle, armed with very strong Thread, through the Basis of the Breast; after which he passed another to cross with the former; then tying the four Ends of the Threads together, it formed a Sort of double Loop, wherewith he suspended the Breast: This being done with a proper Knife contrived to perform the Operation commodiously, he separated the Breast from the Body; after which the Operator made his Ligatures on the Mouths of those divided Arteries which required his Assistance, the Flux of Blood being intirely stopped (which was emitted in continued Streams without any Interruptions) from 4 or 5 Arteries.[165]

After surviving this ordeal, this patient unfortunately died in less than three weeks: her cancer apparently was very aggressive and continued to spread. Beckett considered that the final blow came when the patient sought a cure from 'an old Woman' and used the medications the latter prescribed. These medications, he felt, only made the cancer worse.[166]

Mastectomies carried out with needles and cords were in vogue in the seventeenth and early eighteenth century, but were then gradually discarded. It should be noted, however, that not every seventeenth-century surgeon used the needle and cord technique; some resorted to their hands alone. Wiseman, writing in the latter part of the seventeenth century, clearly epitomized the future shift which would relinquish the cord. He suggested that the surgeon had two options: using either a ligature (the cord), or one's hand to draw the breast. Wiseman himself used a ligature when he amputated.[167] The scalpel and the surgeon's hand took the place of the gruesome needle and cord.

There were several reasons for abandoning this technique. First, there were simpler ways of operating. Boulton, for example, considered his technique to be far simpler and no more difficult than thrusting the cords into the breast: 'the Patient being placed in a convenient Light, the Operator is to pull the Breast to him with one Hand, whilst he cuts it off with the other; and the Flux of Blood is to be stopped with pulv. Galen'.[168] If the cancer – or the breast – was large enough, it was possible to hold it in position without extra devices such as cords. Pierre Dionis also suggested that removing the breast was not particularly difficult for a surgeon:

> The Chirurgeon cuts at the mark'd Place, and takes off the whole Body of the Breast in a short time: This Operation is easier than is imagined before 'tis performed; for the Breast separates as easily from the Ribs, as when we divide the shoulder from a quarter of Lamb.[169]

It may seem shocking at first that Dionis compares removing a human breast to the severing of a lamb carcass; but we should not read this as unfeeling or cold towards the patient. It is rather a comparison in the homely language of the kitchen, understood by all. Actually, it is striking how considerate and empathetic Dionis and his colleagues are throughout. Here, in fact, we come to the second agent of change in the technique of carrying out a mastectomy. I consider it plausible that the gradual rejection of the needle and the ligature was indeed based in part on reasons of empathy for the patient. La Vauguion makes this clear: he was in favour of the new (Helvetian) forceps and 'a crooked knife' and against the use of the cords because they were 'too cruel' for the patient.[170]

Thirdly, the change was facilitated by the availability of new instruments. Forceps had been a great novelty of seventeenth-century breast cancer surgery. Another was the clamp.[171] This device was attached to the breast; it was considered safe, and – particularly important – allowed a quick cutting of the breast. Undoubtedly the patient's safety and comfort, and the avoidance of suffering as far as possible, were important factors in introducing these new ideas. These were aspects that were mentioned when surgeons discussed the patient's position during an operation: whether she should be seated upright, seated in a reclining position, or recumbent. In eighteenth-century surgical tracts this question received much attention; arguably, the discussion was concerned mainly with the comfort of the surgeon, allowing him to carry out the operation safely, quickly and with as little harm to the patient as possible. All these positions had their supporters.[172]

While some significant changes took place in breast cancer surgery in the late seventeenth and early eighteenth century, it was the late eighteenth century that saw something of a revolution. One radical innovation was the closing of the wound immediately after the operation, which radically lessened the time the patient needed to recover from an operation. At this time, what we might call early radical mastectomy was also gaining popularity.

Right after the diseased breast was removed and the blood vessels secured, the teguments were to be brought together. The idea was to cure the wound by covering the wound with skin, and not waiting for a large scab to form.[173] The new technique was seen as especially favourable to the patient. The old technique, for instance, left an ugly scar, since the skin never grew back if the wound was left open: 'the cutis vera is never regenerated; and when destroyed ... the parts under-neath are afterwards covered with thin scarf-skin only'.[174] Undeniably healing was faster with the new technique. Closing the wound 'at first intention' had other benefits for the patient besides faster healing. It saved skin; by cutting away too much skin, Bell noted, 'much unnecessary pain is produced; a very extensive and very ugly sore is left'.[175] This technique had its influence on cutting as well. Saving skin became important. Samuel Sharp noted that 'a longitudinal Incision will dilate sufficiently for the Operation', and recommended that oval cuts be used only on large tumours, and that in amputations it was similarly important to save as much skin as possible.[176] To close the wound, the surgeon could use adhesive plasters or ligatures. Bell preferred ligatures: 'nothing retains the parts so properly in their situation as ligatures; and the pain which they excite is too trifling to be mentioned'.[177]

De Moulin notes that the first surgeon to attempt surgery closing the wound immediately after an operation was a Berlin empiric operating in 1698. The wound was large, and he closed it with five stitches. His patient, however, later died because her cancer spread.[178] De Moulin suggests that this first attempt was important for the subsequent debate as to whether one should indeed try and close the wound and abandon the centuries-old practice.[179] In Britain, the practice of closing the wound gained popularity during the latter part of the eighteenth century, and was at that time clearly considered a radical way of con-cluding the operation. The good results it gave, however, made it popular. Among the proponents of this new technique, and possibly the agent of its introduction into the surgical practice of the 1790s, was the surgeon Henry Fearon, who in the third edition of *A Treatise on Cancers* (1790) was now certain that closing a wound as soon as possible was by far the best way to operate:

> From the further experience of five years, since the publication of the second edition, I am now fully convinced, that the disease is much less liable to return, when the parts have been united by the first intention, than when the operation has been performed in the old way; in which the whole breast was frequently swept off, with too little regard to the sufferings of the patients, and none at all to the preservation of skin.[180]

Fearon, in fact, considered this technique to have been introduced by himself,[181] but in fact it had already been introduced in Britain by the French surgeon Garengeot, whose *A Treatise of Chirurgical Operations* was published in English in 1723.

As already noted, closing the wound at 'the first intention' carried benefits for the patient. It helped the wound to heal more rapidly, dressings were less painful when the operated part was covered by skin and the scar – though still undeniably ugly – was much smaller and less horrible.[182] What further facilitated the acceptance of the technique – which was afterwards also recommended for other amputating operations, such as castration – was the fact that it was not significantly more difficult than the traditional one.[183] When in 1789 John Hunter operated on Miss Worthington's breast and the wound was immediately closed, it came as no great surprise that it healed well, except for a small area which refused to heal. This Hunter accounted for by Miss Worthington's inward weakness after her loss of blood, several ounces in fact, during the operation.[184] Rather than the closing of the wound, the point that interested Hunter in this case was the effect of loss of blood, suggesting that the immediate closure of the wound was by now rather a common procedure.[185] Robert White, in 1796, considered it a new technique which had lately proven superior to the old maxim of leaving the wound open.[186] His view projects a general acceptance of this invention.

This technique required that no extra skin be removed. Benjamin Bell explained that '[i]n every chirurgical operation it should be an established maxim to save as much sound skin as possible. Such portions of the common teguments as are diseased, or that adhere firmly to the parts below, ought certainly to be taken away; but it can never be proper to remove more than this.' Only when a cancer was very advanced – which happened more often than Bell wished – was the surgeon to remove skin extensively.[187]

Alongside the trend towards closing the wound at first intention, mastectomies became increasingly daring. In many cases the operation was extended to the lymph nodes and underlying muscle tissue as well. This process was probably encouraged by the growing number of breast amputations; these not only added to practical experience but showed that patients could survive even the most extensive operations, and suggested that their expected life span after the operation was longer if surgeons were thorough.

Radical mastectomy is attributed to William Halsted (in 1882). I suggest, however, we use the term 'early radical mastectomy' to describe these early mastectomies, which included removal of the lymph nodes in the armpits and at least parts of the chest muscle (in practice parts of the *pectoralis major* were removed). The difference compared to Halsted's operation is perhaps only nominal: Halsted removed all of the chest muscle (both *pectoralis major* and *pectoralis minor*).[188]

It should be kept in mind that throughout the early modern period it was already common practice for all cancerous substance to be removed in an operation. It was the extent of the operation which seems to have turned more radical towards the turn of the nineteenth century. Earlier, as already discussed, the general attitude was against extensive operations because if a cancer had spread it was considered altogether futile to operate – if a cancer was well advanced, the patient was considered to have no chance of survival. Early radical mastectomy sprang from the observation that cancer in the breast spread rapidly if the underlying muscle was left intact in the operation. Now it was thought possible to operate on a cancer which had already spread; in such cases, however, all tumours, even the most minute ones, had to be removed. (We should bear in mind that the cell had not yet been 'discovered'.) Emptying the armpit of the lymph nodes could be performed in many ways, with a hook or by making an incision in the armpit and cutting with a scalpel:

> when the glands in the armpit are enlarged, although they might frequently be pulled out either separately or connected together by a hook insinuated below the sound skin at the sore in the breast; yet it answers the purpose better, to lay the glands first bare by an incision in the manner I have advised, and then to dissect them cautiously out with the scalpel. In the course of the dissection, a good deal of assistance may be obtained from passing a strong ligature through the largest gland; by which the whole cluster with which it is connected may be elevated from the parts below, so as to admit of their being more easily cut out with the scalpel; and it often happens, that these indurated glands, run so near to the axillary artery, as to render it highly proper to use every probable means for rendering the dissection safe and easy.[189]

Among the first British surgical treatises to discuss the removal of at least parts of the pectoral muscle was written by William Beckett. His *New Discoveries Relating to the Cure of Cancers* was first published as early as 1711, and was reprinted with additions in 1712 (this is the version used here). Beckett notes that earlier it had been important not to touch the pectoral muscle when amputating a breast, but he suggests that this might in fact be wrong: 'we have seen a very remarkable Case of this Nature, where a Part of that Muscle was cut away, and the Cartilages of Two of the Ribs laid bare, and the Patient happen'd to be cur'd.'[190]

Others returned to the issue years later. Benjamin Gooch supported this idea, and noted that he had 'seen good consequences from such practice', and that it was advisable to cut off a 'considerable' portion.[191] In mid-century Coventry, Wilmer operated radically on two of his breast cancer patients, removing part of the pectoral muscle as well.[192] It is not quite clear whether Pearson included the removal of the parts of the pectoral muscle in what he termed 'the subjacent parts' but it is probable that he did. He wrote that an operation could be carried out even if a tumour had adhered, if it was possible to remove all the surfaces the cancer adhered to.[193] Bernard Peyrilhe without a shadow of a doubt meant the pectoral muscle. For him saving the pectoral muscle made no sense if the cancer could be conquered with such an operation:

> But the danger from the wound when compared with the certainty of death, ought to moderate our fears, with respect to the amputation of the pectoral muscles, &c. even though we should be obliged to carry the amputation as far as the ribs: nor should we despair of the recovery of the patient, even though some portion of the roots of the tumour should remain; provided we are careful to keep off, or at least, to moderate, the inflammation.[194]

To demonstrate the widespread use of early radical mastectomy we can turn to Henry Fearon, who, in reporting on a case in 1790, nonchalantly noted that a patient's pectoral muscle had to be partially removed and two of her ribs laid bare.[195] It is clear that cancer in the breast was now treated with radical methods so often and routinely that it probably no longer raised many eyebrows.

A great number of women survived these operations. How was this possible? Why did they not succumb to bleeding? Why did they not die more often of post-operational sepsis? Their survival was due more to the surgeon's experience-derived skill than to luck, since there were ways to prevent bleeding and inflammation. Heister, for example, used a homely means which he had learnt from Hélvetius: dressings were soaked with a quart of beer, heated, with an ounce of butter. This, Heister noted, was 'of great use in preventing inflammations'.[196] After the operation, bleeding was the worst danger that immediately came to mind as a life-threatening risk. Careful bandaging was thus important, as was the application of various salves to prevent the bandages from damaging the wound.[197] These horrifying operations were survivable.

3 WOMEN'S AGENCY AND ROLE IN CHOICE OF TREATMENT

On discovering a lump in their breast, women were faced with a series of decisions to make and actions to take, and these choices, and the mindsets behind them, will be the focus of the current chapter. Women made choices about the lump: sometimes they decided to ignore it; sometimes they were determined to deal with it quickly. I argue that women were active agents in their own lives, including illness, and that they made their own decisions regarding their treatment. I therefore take a glance at the sources of information on breast cancer that women had available in making such decisions. I also look at the role played in the illness and its treatment by friends, family, neighbours and various medical practitioners. The chapter concludes with a discussion of the attitudes held by patients towards the most drastic of measures and often their last recourse, surgical operation.

The past two decades in the study of women's history have revealed that within the limits of their society and culture, early modern women were active agents in their own lives and prepared for all kinds of challenges. They are no longer seen as merely victims of the patriarchal hegemony: they could run businesses, sign petitions, invest in public buildings, and hold parish and civic office.[1] Similarly, gender history has taken a look at the ways in which both men and women negotiated the conditions of their everyday lives. In her study on gender in the *Athenian Mercury*, Helen Berry explores a fundamental question: 'In what conditions, for example, did men and women appropriate, enact, or test the boundaries of, their prescribed roles?'[2] It has become obvious that these boundaries were much wider and much more flexible than was earlier assumed. Similarly, we can now see that women's bodies were looked at in many lights, and we can see their many shades, not only as objects but also as subjects.[3]

In the following, I look at these subjects, at active agents, who often searched for a cure with great determination when they discovered a small kernel or lump in their breast.[4] Following others, I argue that in becoming a patient the sufferer did not compromise her independence.[5] Far from being ignorant, early modern women were knowledgeable about cancer in the breast. The woman who had a lump in her breast made sure that she knew what she wanted and how to treat her cancerous condition. She had many different sources of information about lumps and their prospects. These sources included their own previous knowledge; books, ranging from recipe collections to religious treatises and from medical to historical studies; information networks of friends and fellow sufferers; and medical practitioners, in the broadest sense of the term.

Women's Knowledge

People knew about tumours, their symptoms and their dangers. As we have seen, it was important to consider any tumour as a potential danger; for a woman who found a lump in her breast, differentiating between different types of tumours was not her first priority. The lump always indicated potential deadliness, which – especially if painful and growing – had to be dealt with one way or another. For many, like the writer Jane Barker, the initial thought was cancer.

Barker, a writer, poet and novelist (1652–1732) wrote a letter to the Augustinian Prioress at Bruges, Mother Theresa (Lady Lucy Herbert) in 1730. The letter begins with apologies for sending 'so od a present' to Mother Theresa.[6] The present was a tumour: 'a cancer which came out of my brest'. She explains the history of the tumour:

> The first appearance of it was in form of a grein of oatmeal, with great iching [*sic*] and between whiles, pricking and shooting, by which Symptoms I knew it to be a cancer, and therefore looked upon it as a death's head, and so resolved to let it work its will, or rather the will of God, only address'd my prayers to our holy King, touching it with his blood, which I had on a little rag, but instead of deminishing, it grew to the bigness you see, which was in the space of some years, still iching [*sic*] and pricking by fits. At last it seem'd to put its head out (as it were) from under its little mole-hill, by degrees put out farther, till its whole vile body came quite out, hanging by a little string like a white thred, of which there are divers witnesses, in particular my little neece, and Coll. Connocks neece, and my fa. confessor. Some perswaded me to clip it off, but I did not, but left as God had disposed it, at last I found it brake off itself, in my bed, no soar or any manner of corruption appearing, but the part perfectly well.[7]

Barker explained that her cancer was extracted miraculously with the powers of the king's blood. She had touched the cancerous part with a rag in which there was some of his blood. As a Jacobite, and a convert to Catholicism, it was for her both a religious and a political mission to send to the English Catholic nuns this great evidence of James's holy status. Barker asserts that her body rid itself of the tumour with the help of the holy king; she interpreted this as a divine intervention, an act of God through his anointed king James.[8]

In the quotation cited above, Barker refers to her tumour as cancer. She knew, because it was common knowledge, that if a lump grew and gave pain it very likely was cancer. As her biographer Kathryn King notes, there is not much evidence that Barker was more knowledgeable about medicine than elite women of her time in general, but this alone meant a great deal of medical skill. She sold her own gout plaster.[9] Barker's interest in anatomy may have been one reason why she decided to keep her tumour and send it to nuns. While Barker herself admitted it was an odd present, it was not altogether unusual to keep tumours after they were removed. Two of Melmoth Guy's patients, Mrs Coleman from Odiam, Hampshire, and Mrs Shaw, a Quaker from Tottenham, kept – at least according to him – their extracted tumours 'in a large bottle of spirits'.[10] A tumour was a proper curiosity in an age which so loved them.

As we saw from the quotation above, Barker was determined about her diagnosis: she *knew* it was cancer because of its appearance and the symptoms it produced in her. She knew there was not much hope – she saw the cancer as the death's head – and decided to leave the tumour alone: she 'resolved to let it work its will, or rather the will of God'. She does not say whether she ever considered consulting a surgeon, but she clearly did not quite remain passively submissive either, as she sought the king's blood as a remedy.

A similar determination can be found in Barker's contemporary and fellow-author Mary Astell (1666–1731).[11] She kept her disease privy to herself, treated herself, and only when she considered it absolutely necessary did she decide to have her breast amputated.[12] To describe her decision, her biographer Ballard is our best source.[13] Ballard describes Astell as a woman in complete control of her body and of what was done to it, treating herself until she very rationally decides that it is time to cut the diseased breast off.

To be able to make decisions like Barker's or Astell's, one needed knowledge and understanding of cancer, even a familiarity with its nature. This knowledge could be obtained from various sources, not the least of these being women's silent knowledge, the force of tradition, which merged with their everyday experience and made recognizing a lump as a possible cancer nearly self-evident. Like Jane Barker and Mary Astell, women could read many symptoms of cancer in the breast. A growing lump and 'pricking pain' told a tale.

Medical knowledge was women's knowledge, in very concrete terms, far into the seventeenth century and beyond.[14] Recipes were part of what was considered a feminine world. Well into the seventeenth century it was a self-evident fact that women mastered medicine-making and distilling; it was only in the eighteenth century that this task was taken over by apothecaries. Perry suggests that this kind of medicalization reflected a change in women's self-image, that there was 'a growing feeling among women that they no longer controlled their own bodies, no longer believed they could understand their own physiological processes, no longer believed in their shared medical and herbal knowledge, no longer expected to exercise independent judgment about how to deploy their bodies'.[15] Women certainly gave up some of their previous medical activities, but Perry's picture may still be overly pessimistic as a description of the eighteenth-century situation. Women were not excluded from the discussion when it came to their bodies. While medical knowledge did become increasingly pro-fessionalized towards the end of the century, women still made the decisions that concerned their bodies – and even though they sometimes scorned women's medical activities, medical practitioners at times still used women's knowledge to their advantage.[16] Thus it is only logical to assume that women too used their own knowledge as a first resort.

Hannah Murray's account of her diagnosed breast cancer speaks of the acceptance of women's knowledge in treating a cancer. John Patterson wrote down her account in 1745 and published it in 1763. We have little reason to doubt that the main points of this account were as she told them – he took it 'from her mouth'. Hannah Murray was twenty-two when a 'blue speck, about the bigness of a corn of gunpowder' appeared on her left breast. She had it for seven years, and suffered some pain before there appeared a lump in the breast which grew to the size of an egg in a few weeks:

> Then taking the advice of the most skilful surgeons, who concluded it was a cancer of the worst sort; I was directed to a gentlewoman that had been cured of a cancer, whose directions I followed, and, with a blessing on the means, I obtained a cure. She directed me to take the leaves and small branches of Pokeweed, pound them together, and squeeze the juice, put it into an earthen pot, and set it in the sun, until it acquired the thickness of an ointment, then spread a plaster on the leaf of a plant, no bigger than the knot (the leaf was to be used when green, in the winter black silk) and to apply a new plaster four or five times in 24 hours, if I could endure the pain, which was exceeding sharp: she told me it would make it apparently worse, for it would draw it to the outside from the bottom, which I found to be true; for in a small time after I used the means, it opened five holes in my breast, the biggest where the speck was, which was big enough to put in the end of the my thumb. She told me to take no physic, nor use any strong drink, except in case of faintness; which means I used from August to March, and then it healed on a sudden, and hath been well now twelve years.[17]

Hannah Murray's account suggests that she had seen surgeons who diagnosed her condition as cancer, decided there was nothing they could do and so directed her to see the gentlewoman who had herself been cured of cancer. This gentle-women ordered Murray a strong caustic medicine, which in the end cured her. Pokeweed (*Phytolacca Americana*) is a highly poisonous plant, which inciden-tally is still used and researched as a cancer medicine. While we cannot be certain that it was the surgeons who directed Murray to see the gentlewoman, as the formulation does not make it clear who it was, the triumph of the account is the gentlewoman's: using her means she was able to cure the patient, something the surgeons could not accomplish. By publishing this detailed account of the pro-cess of the cure, John Patterson advanced women's experience and knowledge to his medical colleagues in a professional publication. As Murray's case shows, women's expertise even in such poisonous herbal medications as pokeweed was acceptable, and it was only very slowly that male learned culture came to dominate botany[18] – if it ever did so in everyday practice. The fact that elite women ceased preparing their medicines in their distilling houses did not mean that they gave up their family recipes: they merely bought their favourite medications ready-made, and added to their lists some new chemical medications as well. This may well explain the long-lived popularity of certain easily home-made breast cancer medications.[19] A good example of one such is the plaster made of goose dung and celandine. The recipe was very popular in the sixteenth and seventeenth centuries, but was proposed for use on breast cancer in 1770. It can be found in *The Treasure of Pore Men* in 1526:

> Take ye fenne of a Geyte & the ioyce of Celodyne & myngle them togyder & lay it on the sore[20]

In 1631 it appeared in A.T.'s *A Rich Storehouse*:

> Take Goose-dung and Celendine, bray them well together, and lay it on the Canker two nights.[21]

In 1653 it was recommended by the anonymous author of *A Book of Fruits & Flowers*:

> Take Goose-dung, and Celedonie, stamp them well together, and lay it plaister wise to the soare, it will cleanse the *canker*, kill the wormes, and heale the soare.[22]

Twenty years later, Hannah Woolley's compilations, *The Gentlewomans Companion* (1673) and *The Accomplish'd Lady's Delight* (1675), cited the same remedy, the first being almost identical to the earlier one:

> Take Goos-dung and Cellydony, stamp them well together, and lay them Plaisterwise on the sore; this shall cleanse the Cancer, kill the Worm, and heal the Sore.[23]

The latter presented the same recipe in a slightly different formula:

> Take The Dung of a Goose, and the Juice of Celandine, and bray them well in a Mortar together, and lay it to the Sore, and this will stay the Cancer, and heal it.[24]

And in 1770, Catherine Brooks listed it in *The Complete English Cook* for a cancer in the breast:

> [A]pply Goose Dung and Celandine beat well together, and spread on a fine Rag; it will both cleanse and heal the Sore.[25]

This medication was not difficult to prepare. Goose dung was readily available, and the juice of celandine was a popular medication for other medical problems as well.[26] Recipes for treating cancers in popular handbooks were numerous, clearly reflecting the wealth of material in women's and families' own recipe books.[27]

Manuscript recipe collections[28] were often women's creations and in women's use, used within a family for a lengthy period of time, and passed on to daughters and granddaughters or other members of the family. And, naturally, recipes were shared. These collections show that women often had excellent resources even at home to start treating their breast problems, and to advise others. A good example of such a book is the Temple family collection of household and medical recipes, which was in use for a long period of time, probably from the mid-seventeenth to the mid-eighteenth century.[29] This collection includes a poultice for breasts and a medicated dressing for an ulcerated breast cancer, attributed to the great surgeon William Chiselden.[30]

The fact that these collections included well-known breast cancer remedies does not give us automatic licence to assume that the recipes were ever used; but the inclusion of breast cancer remedies in such collections suggests that cancer was a disease for which one wanted to have a remedy available, just in case. The Eyton collection, in use from the late seventeenth century until at least 1738, suggests an illness within the close circle of the users of the collection.[31] In the case of the Arscott collection it is known that Mrs Arscott was the sufferer.[32] The manuscript contains a separate leaf, possibly written by a physician or a surgeon, depicting part of the course of her illness. This leaf describes the trials Mrs Arscott went through with bark (probably Peruvian), a popular medicine for cancer, from December 1742 to the end of May 1743. She was treated by a Mr Ranby, who had had good results with bark 'on Two or Three'. She was asked not to omit other medications, and it seems likely that she might have been using opiates at the time, pointing towards an advanced and painful stage of the illness. The bark did not change her situation at all, nor did it 'lessen her pain nor abate the discharge', which reveals that her breast had ulcerated. By Mr Ranby's advice, Mrs Arscott gave up the bark because it had no effect. She remained very ill but improved in the spring: there was less discharge and it was thicker, and 'many parts seemed healing, the pain inconsiderable to what it had been, her appetite good, & her spirits Free & easy'. She wanted to return to the bark, believing it was the cause of her improved health, but her symptoms returned, and indeed in May they became 'as violent as ever'.[33]

Several recipes recorded in the collection are ascribed to specific women. This does not necessarily mean that these recipes were always directly given to the collector by the named person, although sometimes they were; but this practice reflects a cultural female trait of sharing medical information, and further foregrounds the importance and great value of women's medical and pharmaceutical knowledge in early modern culture, which continued in the eighteenth century.

The recipes included in the first hundred folios of the Arscott collection were written down for ordinary reasons, for curiosity and perhaps for later use. There is a recipe, for example, for 'Doctor Sydenham's Liquid Laudanum', for a plaister to ease breast swellings and cancers, a plaster for cancer given by a Mr Ball of Honiton, and a recipe for cancer 'recommended by Lady Northampton'. On folio 152 there is another recipe for cancer, a lime drink for a cancer given by Lady Molesworth, and this is soon followed by detailed instructions for a cancer from Mrs Fuller, dated 1739. (Perhaps this focus on breast cancer treatment comes about because at this point Mrs Ascott suspects she has the disease herself.) In addition, the patient is asked to try only foods that are easily digested, such as chicken and veal, and to avoid cheese, French claret and strong beer. The diseased breast should be kept warm and not treated with any irritating medications: Mrs Fuller writes that 'I had a vast many things prescribed me to use outwardly but I never try'd any of them & I hope your friend will not be prevail'd on to anoint or bath ye breast however recomended for it often does great mischief – be sure to observe great Temperance & go very easily Laced.'[34] The wealth of advice here perfectly integrates good and well-tested medications with advice from friends and patients, along with doctors. Typical in this sense is a tip for a diet drink which is attributed to 'the Famous Dr Louther'. Its efficacy had been proved by a Mrs Hales, who was mentioned to the mother of Mrs Wyatt, who had found great relief and cure after she had been 'order'd' to have her breast cut off. Mrs Hales had, it is said, lived no less than thirty years afterwards, 'in Perfect Health'.[35] To live long in perfect health was undoubtedly the great hope of the likes of Mrs Arscott. The range and extent of advice included in the Arscott collection speaks of a desperation to find a cure; but it also reveals that when detected, breast problems were announced to friends and family, a search for remedies was initiated and help was received from many directions. Indeed it seems that the cancer recipes in the last part of the collection are there specifically to help Mrs Arscott. The index to the collection gives further proof: it seems quite final without these cancer medicines, which were added to the index later, in a different hand and a different ink.[36]

A great deal of information about diseases came from the printing press. Already mentioned was the abundance of printed recipe and household books. By the turn of the eighteenth century, women's reading was by no means a matter for the elite classes only. From recent research we now know that girls of the middling sort nearly always had some schooling and so did many girls of the poorer classes. It was possible for a great number of women to read about breast cancer themselves if they so wanted.[37] Since the great majority of medical books, both 'professional' and 'popular', were written in English, they were at least in theory available to all reading women. Roy Porter suggests that the desire to 'enlighten' people and to change their deplorable ways was one important reason why writers so eagerly published in English. Mary Fissell considers the fundamental role these books had 'as entertainment, as memory devices, as statements about man's (and sometimes woman's) relationship to the natural world, and as instructions on how to manipulate that world'.[38]

The power of print was immense in early modern England, and the number of books published in the eighteenth century was staggering. Popular works could be distributed in the thousands and go into dozens of editions, and popular medical books proliferated in the seventeenth century onwards. Specialized books, such as medical self-help books or advice on recipes, did not go unnoticed by potential readers and buyers, who were served in 1700 by some two hundred booksellers in fifty towns.[39] In this sense knowledge was not elitist in nature, and many women were able to own or borrow surgical and medical books which they could consult if they, or anyone close to them, found a lump in their breast. Having said that, however, one has to once again recognize that literary information was only one kind of reliable information available. Women did rely on other sources as well; knowledge was not as hierarchical as we tend to think. Recent research has suggested that there was a tendency to move from the oral tradition to the printed word in the search for information, and from women's knowledge to the printed (male) word in seeking answers to questions pertaining to women's matters.[40] This reflects the slow but ongoing process of the professionalization of medical care in general.

In the eighteenth century books were an essential source of information. If one did not want to accumulate a library of one's own, books could be borrowed. Parochial libraries were beginning to appear, and especially significant were commercial circulating libraries, which could add significantly to the corpus of texts women had available. The first such library was founded in 1718 in Huntingdon. Peter Borsay notes that these libraries were especially popular in spa towns such as Bath.[41] For a fixed annual fee, one could subscribe to a library and enjoy a wealth of books when away from home or if one's own library did not include specific medical titles.

John Bell advertised his huge circulating library in London, consisting of more than 50,000 books. His catalogue, however, comprised 8,486 titles. Among the topics covered by his library were history, geography and gardening, as well as physic, surgery and anatomy.[42] His folio-sized books included James's *Medical Dictionary* in three volumes;[43] in quarto he had the *Catalogue of Simple Medicines that are Fit to be Used in the Practice of Physick and Surgery*, Heister's *Medical, Chirurgical and Anatomical Cases* and Macbride's *Introduction to Physic*.[44] Bell also stocked a number of octavo-sized medical treatises, including Dr Allen's three-volume *Synopsis Medicinæ*, Astruc's *Diseases of Women with Child*, several works by Boerhaave, Bromfield's *Observations and Cases in Surgery* (including volume one, which discussed amputation, tumours etc.), *Dionis's*

Course of Chirurgical Operation, Hill's *Cases in Surgery,* Maubray's *Female Physician,* the *Memoirs of the Academy of Surgery at Paris,* in two volumes, one of which dealt with cancers; Sharpe's treatises on surgery, Turner's two-volume *The Art of Surgery,* and Vanswieten's treatise on Boerhaave in fourteen volumes, of which volume 4 dealt with cancer.[45] While Bell's library may well have been exceptional, circulating libraries in provincial towns were also reasonably well stocked in surgical literature. In 1791, R. Fisher's circulating library in Newcastle held the famous surgeon Benjamin Bell's *System of Surgery* in six volumes, of which volume 5 dealt with tumours, and Albrecht Haller's *Medical, Surgical and Anatomical Cases and Experiments.*[46]

Important information about cancer in the breast was also found in other genres of writing. History taught lessons as well: many women were keen on reading about history, and historical knowledge was passed on through the oral tradition – a moving narrative about famous women, saints and queens who had suffered from the disease could be imprinted on one's memory for a long time.[47]

There were no miracles involved in the illness of Anne of Austria,[48] only horrible suffering, of which many read in the detailed and lengthy biography by Madame de Motteville, first published in English in 1725. Anne of Austria was a famous character, and the general interest in her is not only reflected in the publication of de Motteville's work in English; her life was also discussed elsewhere,[49] and inspired others. For example, after reading de Motteville, the poet Mary Barber wrote about the life of the former Queen of France. Perhaps the end of the series of events which forms the history of Anne of Austria, her horrifying death from breast cancer, inspired awe in Barber:

> Reflect, my Soul, that Day is drawing near;
> And timely think, what was thy Business here.
> O Thou, whose Arm, reach'd down from Heav'n to save,
> So lately snatch'd me from the op'ning Grave;
> Who bow'd thine Ear, nor let me sue in vain,
> Reliev'd my Sickness, and remov'd my Pain;
> In hallow'd Strains, O, teach my Soul to soar,
> To celebrate the Mercies I adore!
> To Thee alone to dedicate my Lays,
> Who heard my Vows, and added to my Days!
> Watch o'er my Heart, fix ev'ry Duty there,
> And make Eternity my only Care.[50]

De Motteville's account of the dowager Queen's illness is long and dramatic; the modern reader finds it hair-raising at times, as it delves into Anne's overwhelming pains and the long-lasting anguish caused by her cancer.

An English woman reading Anne's *Memoirs* in the eighteenth century, if she had the stomach to read the fifth volume, had quite a reading experience before her. Disturbing to the modern reader, in the eighteenth century de Motteville's history of Anne's illness must have been imposing reading with its ninety pages of Anne's sufferings. In her account de Motteville presents images of a woman torn by the factions of the court, of desperate but useless physicians and of the king's varied moods towards his mother and his express wishes for her treatment. Similarly, I argue below, most sufferers turned very early after the onset of their symptoms to their friends, family and neighbours for help and advice, arguably signifying a great degree of openness.

Secrets?

This openness is contrary to my initial thinking. Some of the first sources I found on breast cancer – here Mary Astell was especially important – seemed to suggest that women wanted to keep their tumours secret until it was utterly impossible to conceal their condition. This, I thought, would be for two main reasons: first, a tumour was frightening and it would have been easier to ignore it; and secondly, breasts were part of the sexual body, which it was inappropriate to reveal, especially to men.

Such a consultation may have been difficult for many, since chastity and modesty walked hand in hand in the eighteenth century, forming a cultural norm. It had been the case since ancient days. In his *Life of St Macrina*, Gregory of Nyssa pointed out that his sister Macrina, who suffered from an ulcerated breast cancer, was cured of her wound by the will of God. This happened through her own tears, which fell on the ground and mixed with earth; she took this mud and applied it to the sore. This, together with her mother's sign of the Holy Cross on her bosom, miraculously healed her. The important teaching in this history was not only that Macrina escaped the surgeon's knife, but especially that she saved her chastity by not having to show her breast to the surgeon, a man: 'she judged it worse than the pain, to uncover any part of the body to a stranger's eyes'.[51] This avoidance seems to have been a commonplace notion in antiquity, where, as Helen King posits, women were 'prevented both from knowing what [was] wrong with them, and from speaking to a *iatros* if they [did] know, by their youth, inexperience and embarrassment'.[52] In the Middle Ages, *The Trotula* stated: 'women, from the condition of their fragility, out of shame and embarrassment do not dare reveal their anguish over their diseases (which happen in such a private place) to a physician'.[53] This sense of shame is a prolonged trend in history. Indeed, Susan Sontag has argued that in the twentieth century cancer was still perceived as embarrassing and shameful.[54]

Eighteenth-century women often had to make a different decision to Macrina's, and at some point needed a male eye to judge and diagnose their cancers; but they often waited a long time before resorting to that. In this procrastination, modesty certainly played a part: some women were reluctant to talk about their cancers to others, to anyone. As mentioned, Mary Astell seems to have managed her breast cancer in secret for a long time, perhaps even several years, before she decided to have a mastectomy. Her biographer George Ballard wrote in 1752:

> She seemed to enjoy an uninterrupted state of health 'till a few years before her death, when, having one of her breasts cut off, it so much impaired her constitution, that she did not long survive it. This was occasioned by a cancer, which she had concealed from the world in such a manner, that even few of her most intimate acquaintance knew any thing at all of the matter. She dressed and managed it herself, 'till she plainly perceived there was an absolute necessity for its being cut off.[55]

According to Ballard, Astell asked Mr Johnson to take the breast 'off in the most private manner imaginable'.[56] Perhaps her decisions about the operation were ruled by modesty; this would be a logical explanation for her insistence that no extra persons should attend her operation. Ballard notes how she 'would hardly allow him [Mr Johnson] to have persons whom necessity required to be at the operation'.[57] More than modesty, however, it is possible that, being a person of some fame, she did not want the public to know of her ordeal and illness; that she considered these to be private matters.

It is impossible to say what exactly Richard Guy meant when he wrote that a patient of his who 'had a Scirrhus in the Breast, which she had imprudently kept to herself' until it was life-threatening.[58] Did she really not tell anyone about the tumour? Or did she not see doctors, but talked about the lump to friends and family? Either way, in Guy's opinion she reacted too late. Even though great efforts were put into her cure, the cancer apparently spread (according to Guy to her liver) and she died. Guy mentions that he had known many such cases, and writes that it would be tautological to go through them.[59] It is thus possible that such cases were more frequent than the surviving evidence actually shows; that women did not want to see doctors, and that they were especially reluctant to consult surgeons, seems to emerge as a general perception. Perhaps some women kept their lumps secret from their family as long as possible in order not to be pressured into consultations with medical practitioners. At second glance, however, the fact that women did not seek a surgeon's help the very moment they realized they might have a tumour in their breast does not necessarily mean that they were actively hiding it. Rather, I suggest, they were waiting, hoping for the lump to disappear (without the need for surgery), and – as we have already seen – seeking for relief elsewhere and by different methods.

Perhaps surprisingly, this kind of secrecy does not declare itself in more prominent terms in eighteenth-century texts. Of course, if there were women who kept silent (if indeed there were many of them), and if they were successful, they did not necessarily end up in books. It is unlikely, however, that many managed such secrecy for very long. Most women spoke to someone of their concern about a lump quite early on. For most women, I argue, diseases in general were shared; they simply did not necessarily share their worries with a physician or surgeon as soon as these professionals would have wanted them to. This is most likely why many medical professionals ended up thinking that women were too timid and ashamed to relate their health problems to them in time to save lives.[60] Below I discuss further the idea which seemed to prevail, in particular among surgeons, that women were too timid to resort to the knife at a very early stage, or at least at an early enough stage. Many practitioners who wanted to hurry their patients into their care felt frustration at patients' reluctance to rely solely on them.

This is not to argue that women were not modest, or that they would not have found it difficult to consult a male practitioner. Modesty was a cultural norm, and the way in which male surgeons had to exhort ladies into acting contrary to the feminine role is interesting.[61]

Modern Family Physician (1775) urged its readers not to wait, and attested that

> Many persons, especially women, endeavour to conceal it [cancer] too long, and so prevent medicines having their proper effects, whereas had it been taken in time all these evils would have been remedied, and the disorder itself removed before it arose to an incurable height.[62]

The author's claim that it was women in particular who waited too long with their cancers arguably suggests an association with chastity and patient procrastination, but this could have pointed towards women's general modesty as well. Richard Guy wrote explicitly that women often concealed their cancer because of 'Delicacy'.[63]

But we should keep in mind that secrecy and modesty are two different matters. It thus remains highly possible that many women did not necessarily want to keep their tumours secret, but preferred to consult other women or their friends only and to avoid the male gaze.[64]

As I have discussed elsewhere[65] the role women's friendships and networks in finding a cure for breast cancer, we won't delve into these questions here. Suffice it to say that women were dependent on their social circles, their families and their elite sponsors when looking for help.

Friends were needed at the consultation as well. The diagnosis was customarily discussed with the patient's friends and family; sometimes – though probably only exceptionally – friends were the first to hear the verdict, while the patient was informed later.[66] If this was the case, it was in order to ask the patient's friends for advice on how best to break the news to her, and to allow them to soften the blow. This, once again, does not support the idea that cancer was conscientiously hidden. Cancer was not a secret matter. Illness could be shared by vast circles such as in the case of Mrs Evans, from Grange Street in Southwark, who had a large tumour in her breast when she consulted 'an eminent surgeon'. This surgeon suggested she have her breast operated on, but Mrs Evans refused because she dreaded 'so painful an operation'. The surgeon (Burrows) apparently managed to cure her by other means, and suggests that her Quaker brethren and her neighbours were emotionally involved in her illness. Speaking of her perfect recovery in his care, her surgeon notes that

> she was perfectly restored, to her own unspeakable pleasure, and the surprize of many of her brethren and neighbours, who implicitly relying on the opinion of some of the faculty, had intimated, that her case was beyond her power of medicine, and to be remedied but by extirpation alone.[67]

Without doubt women also turned to their menfolk for help. The evidence shows that many fathers and husbands were deeply involved in finding a cure and taking care of the patient. Alexander Morgan had a twenty-three-year-old patient, a maid, whom he cured of her breast problems. It was the girl's father who 'discharged' Morgan when her tumour had disappeared, after a series of treatments lasting for several months. As she came to see him from the country, it is quite probable that her father accompanied her to town to see Morgan. She was not present when he was dismissed. Morgan notes the role of the father in finding out about the patient's situation: 'her father told me that ye tumoer was quite gon but they did strictly observe to Respect boath ye Eleect & ye purge as it was about prescribed'.[68] Interestingly, the treatment is a matter of *their* doing; it was not only the patient's responsibility, but seems to have involved her family and especially her father as well. This does not speak only of the young woman's dependent position in the world, but also of emotional attachment and caring. It also reflects the importance of the feared disease: it was worth it for the parents and others to become involved in the course of treatments. The vital goal was to find a cure for a probably fatal tumour. Many husbands, such as Mordecai Cary whose fears I have explored elsewhere,[69] were closely involved in attempts to cure their wives' illness. An illness as grave as cancer in the breast commonly moved a multitude of people into action.

Medical Practitioners

Next, let us take a look at the role given by women with breast cancer to physicians and surgeons. As we have seen, their role in curing breast cancers was not as immediate and central as it is today, now that cancer is seen as a disease requiring instant oncological attention. What help could physicians and surgeons offer in the long eighteenth century? Nowadays, for the overwhelming majority of us, it is a given that we seek a doctor's advice if there seems to be anything very wrong with our health. There is a whole army of medical professionals whom we can consult, and who we believe possess a certain kind of knowledge unavailable to us as laypersons. The status of medicine in eighteenth-century England was not yet such, although the prominence of the medical profession was growing. Its requirement of a university education (although not necessarily in medicine) gave the profession its high status, but it held no monopoly in medical matters.[70]

In problems of the breast, it would be logical to expect that especially women of child-bearing age would first contact a midwife for help. Mrs Hays of Wilton did just that, when a lump grew rapidly within a few months after she had first perceived it.[71] It is somewhat surprising, however, that Mrs Hays's consultation with a midwife has left a rare trace in the records. This rarity, however, may not reflect the reality, but merely the fact that in listing their patients' previous consultations my sources fail to mention midwives. On the other hand this would be surprising, since they do mention other kinds of help. If this rarity does reflect reality and midwives were only rarely consulted in cases of tumours, it may be that women were themselves easily able to distinguish between a tumour and a milk abscess (for which it would have been natural to seek advice from a midwife) and that they did not direct their questions to midwives when they suspected cancer.

At the end of the day, many women who were desperate about a growth in their breast would consult a surgeon. In many cases they would have consulted a physician first; but traditionally physicians had not been allowed to shed blood, in that as university men they had been clergymen.[72] This division of labour continued down to the seventeenth century, and its effects were still apparent in the eighteenth century. In serious cases such as breast cancer, if a woman needed a mastectomy it would have been a surgeon who performed the operation.[73] Ideally, the patient's physician would have been present, but would not have been involved in the operation.

We have already seen that women in distress turned to all kinds of help, including those who were condemned by university physicians as quacks. From the patient's point of view it made sense to seek help wherever it was available – and many practitioners promised a fast cure. Medical knowledge and quackery were a popular topic for cheap print, which 'supplied a seemingly endless demand for aphrodisiac recipes, potions for barrenness, conditions and signs for conceiving a boy or girl, avoiding miscarriage, and easing labour pains'.[74] It would be interesting to study the opportunities mountebanks had in spreading the awareness of cancers: charlatans would often hold a show to impress his audience with their skills, but those with medical training would greatly disapprove of these practitioners, and wanted to expose them to the general audience.[75] Among the cases which the notorious healer, the Irish Stroker, Valentine Greatrakes, was famed to have cured were 'Cancerous Knots in the Breast'.[76] Cured cancer was a great advertisement for his trade, although he was especially famous for curing the King's Evil (or scrofula) and ague.[77] Henry Stubbe noted that he had begun his stroking with breast cancers and scrofula, and only later added other conditions to his repertoire.[78] His own book contains a number of testimonies to his successes. It seems to show that cancers were not his foremost trade while he was in England, but there is one case which had been deemed to be a cancerous breast. This woman, Dorothy Pocock, says in her (probably dictated) testimony, signed by four witnesses, the following:

> Dorothy the Wife of John Pocock of Chiveley in the County of Berks, aged 45. had a Tumour began in her breast about August 1665. which in the beginning of April 1666. was grown so big as a large Pullets Egge, and conceived by sundry Physitians and Chirurgeons to be a Cancer, and no other way of curing it then by cutting out; was stroked twice by Mr. Greatraks', and after the second time, the Tumour was grown softer, so that he opened it, and out thereof flowed a great quantity of concocted matter; and after that by gentle stroking Mr. Greatrak's brought forth the bag wherein the matter had lyen out of the small orifice; and she professes her self to be very well of her breast, and also to be freed of a great pain which she had in her arm and shoulder for the space of 8 months last past. April 10. 1666. Dorothy Pocock.[79]

This evidence of his using incisions for cancer is in accordance with what Stubbe notes about his technique. Greatrakes, according to him, was 'still a stranger to all Physique and Chirurgery' but had lately started cutting tumours because stroking seemingly was not strong enough to dissolve tumours – it merely ripened some humours.[80]

Mountebanks might have carried with them collections of specimens. Daniel Defoe suggests this possibility in his *The Compleat Mendicant*. Regardless of his earlier enjoyment of his travelling companion, the mendicant despises the man when he finds out he is nothing but a common swindler who specializes in fooling people into believing in his healing skills and potions.[81]

Rowley wrote a long and eloquent piece against quacks who promised a painless cure for cancer. They took advantage of the 'patient's hope and fear'.[82] Mentally, it was perhaps easy for the patient to succumb to treatments that promised a straightforward and quick cure. While the surgeon's craft often promised drastic and painful measures, the physician's skills were in healing in the long term, and they prided themselves in not promising quick cures for cancers. They felt that their own skills, in combination with surgery, had the correct tools for any treatment of cancer, and complained about women's refusal to recognize that a physician was better skilled to treat their breasts than a quack:

> It often happens, however,
> from an improper delicacy in patients,
> as well as from other causes,
> that practitioners are not consulted
> till the disease is far advanced.[83]

It seems to have been a commonplace opinion among physicians and surgeons that patients turned to their help too late. Some of the causes for this have been discussed above. Did women in fact consult them 'late'? It seems indeed that the professionals' experience reflects their patient's ways of shopping for treatment. Many women seem to have sought help from a physician fairly early on, often within the first year of their trouble; they certainly did not consult a physician as soon as the latter would have wished, but they do not seem to have been *against* such consultations. Time was a relative matter; the condition of the breast and the nature of the tumour were much more pressing. Women seem to have acted according to the information their bodies gave them and prompted them to do. Indeed, Janet Kirkpatrick, a thirty-year-old woman, had a tumour for six years, but did nothing about it because there was no pain. When the number of tumours increased, she sought treatment.[84] Or, in another case, Mrs Jennings from Bedfordshire reported in 1814 first noticing her lump some time in 1809. She does not specify the precise date, suggesting that she may not have been certain about it.[85] She had 'thought little' of her lump 'until the spring following',[86] the spring of 1810. It had taken her at least six months before she had began to worry about the lump. It seemed larger than earlier, it was clearly growing and it was becoming more painful. Progress was quite rapid here, as she said in June; the application of leeches gave her some relief.[87] The use of leeches, a normal treatment for a woman of her age, suggests that by June she had consulted a physician or a surgeon.[88]

The case studies of patients that I have come across seem to have taken active decisions about their treatments and the pace of it, regardless of their social status and economic situation. It is possible that the poorer the patient, the longer it took for her to seek expert help; but that is not reflected in my sources. Doctors and surgeons treated poor patients as well. This may seem to be an idealized view, but my sources show no evidence to the contrary. This of course may be due to the nature of the sources, which list only patients who were actually treated. However, even those who had fallen off the society ladder could receive medical attention.[89]

It seems typical that a woman with a lump in her breast sought help from physicians and surgeons when the tumour became painful. Pain was a worrying and alarming sign, not necessarily raised by the more common knot in the breast; it also brought discomfort, which one needed to abate. In general, women were clearly able to tolerate some growth of the lump, but became frightened and distressed when the lump started sending pains: darting, lancing, pricking sensations. Thus, very typically, at the turn of the nineteenth century a lady's maid had watched a tumour grow in her breast for two years, 'but felt no great uneasiness till within the last twelve months; during which period she had daily experienced several severe darting pains, which became more so as the tumour increased'.[90] In the 1760s, Mrs Harley, from Welbeck Street in Marylebone, had sought help from a surgeon at the point when her pain increased daily and she was 'at length unable to rest'.[91]

Help was regularly sought from specialists too, and they could be found especially in London and in Edinburgh. If a case was desperate, London surgeons would receive patients from great distances. Spa towns and, at the end of the century, certain hospitals too developed specialized cancer wards.[92]

Saying No to the Knife

The new cancer wards would offer their patients a chance for surgery as well. This was often the last resort for poor and rich alike, and many abhorred the very thought of surgery. The Frenchman Pierre Dionis had regretted that the surgeon was rarely able to use his knife when the cancer was young and small, and he too reminded his readers that it was best to operate as soon as possible.[93] Buchan noted that 'One misfortune attending the disease is, that the unhappy patient often conceals it too long',[94] and Culpeper's *English Physician* similarly regretted that the patient would not see the knife as a resource until 'till death stares them in the face'.[95] Patients' reluctance may simply suggest a fear of surgery, but it may also reflect a lack of confidence in it; perhaps patients did not consider it worthwhile.

As we saw in Chapter 1, opinions as to the benefits of mastectomies and other surgical procedures varied greatly. It was often recognized that speedy action in the treatment of breast cancer was advisable; but it seems that women were not expected to resort eagerly to the knife, if at all. It was traditionally acceptable to refuse surgery.

It is impossible to know whether the choice not to undergo surgery represented a majority of breast cancer sufferers, but in any case it is safe to assert that there were a great number of women who decided against an operation. The most obvious reason for declining an operation even when it was warmly recommended seems to have been fear. I analyse the emotional side of cancer in Chapter 4; here I focus on the choices women made.

Women's active decisions about their future, even when they were in horrific pain, tormented without a moment's rest, are evident throughout the source material presented throughout this work. It was always ultimately the woman herself who decided whether or not to have her breast amputated, and women often had a clear view of the situation even before they consulted a physician or surgeon. There were also cases where a woman wanted to have an operation but her practitioner opposed it. Ethically too, as Andrew Wear reminds us, it was impossible for a surgeon to press a patient strongly about an operation she did not want to have. Similarly, surgeons could not give false hope regarding the possible success of curing cancer by amputation.[96] Andrew Duncan's *Medical Cases* (1781) for example confirms Wear's notion:

> I had no hesitation in recommending it to this patient to think of operation, and to consult surgeons with respect to it; but I found her totally adverse to all thoughts of it. And I must here observe, that it is an operation attended with so much danger, that I should reckon it improper to go any further than merely to recommend it.[97]

Benjamin Gooch adds an interesting proposition to this: the surgeon should spare the patient's emotions, but be more frank with her family and friends:

> When it appears advisable to propose the operation, we should with prudence and precaution give our opinion concerning the expediency of it, without intimidating the patient with the precariousness of the event; though we should be more explicit in this point to the relations or friends, for our own justification should it not end happily.[98]

When a surgeon, alone or with colleagues, recommended an operation to a patient, they almost certainly gave her or her friends all the medical facts they knew and let the patient decide for herself, even if her decision differed from the recommendations of the learned and experienced. Henry Fearon offers us glimpses of such events in the late eighteenth century, in which two practitioners were trying to persuade a woman with a schirrus to allow them to remove the tumour.[99] Elizabeth Turner had been admitted to the Surrey Dispensary in around 1782.[100] She was a patient of Dr Sims's, but her case came to Fearon's knowledge when Sims consulted him: Sims considered it advisable for Mrs Turner to have surgery, and Fearon agreed. The tumour had been developing for a year and a half; it had no known origin, but was movable and had not adhered to anything, and the glands in her axilla were not enlarged. These were all positive indications of a good outcome for an operation. He and Sims 'accordingly took great pains to recommend' an operation, but it was 'without effect'.[101] Despite their 'great pains', which probably meant quite a strong attempt to persuade the patient, she would not hear of it, and walked out.

Unfortunately, the history of Elizabeth Turner's illness unfortunately does not end in triumph. Sims and Fearon heard from her again a fortnight later, and a great change had taken place. They went to her apartments in the Maze, and found her in a sad state:

> I found her in bed, with her head and shoulders supported; she breathed very quick and with great difficulty, her pulse was quick and small, she was in the most excruciating pain, insomuch that she said she was then ready to have her breast taken off, and would undergo any thing to get relief. In the above short time, the breast had increased considerably, and adhered in every part to the ribs with a firmness that I cannot express. The muscles of the abdomen, neck and arm, on that side, were all enlarged, and contracted, so that her head and thigh were bent towards each other.[102]

Only two weeks had changed her situation dramatically. She had probably left the Dispensary horrified at the surgeons' insistence on her having to lose her breast, but she was now in such pain that she was willing to 'undergo any thing'. The surgeons thought it was now too late for her; Fearon noted that in her 'melancholy situation' not even opium provided any help. Only three days later, 'death put an end to her torture'.[103]

Mary Smith, at forty, was diagnosed with a true schirrus and was recommended an operation. After hearing this she disappeared for two weeks, during which time, according to Fearon, she had seen 'an eminent surgeon' several times. She returned to Fearon, however, now willing to proceed with the removal of the breast. Her breast was now much worse since the tumour had adhered to her pectoral muscle, and there were smaller lumps elsewhere. There was also a greatly enlarged gland in her axilla. Fearon was no longer able to promise much, since 'absorption' had taken place – the illness had spread – and her chances to outlive it were small. But the patient wanted to take any chance she had: 'Her reply was, that she suffered such acute and almost constant pain, that she would run any risk.'[104] Not uniquely, it was pain that drove Mary Smith to the decision to give up her breast.

Elizabeth Benham of Prospect-Row, Walworth, waited ten years before finally consenting to an operation. She had refused surgery because 'she suffered no inconvenience, except from its weight, and at times a dull heavy pain' but as the tumour gradually grew and her pains increased she consulted Sims; he advised her to have her breast removed by Fearon, and she finally readily consented. Her wound healed so quickly that she was able to walk only days after her surgery.[105] Fearon had earlier tried to persuade Mrs Benham by arguing that no one could tell how long the tumour would remain silent, and that it was less painful to operate at an early stage than at an advanced one, but she had refused. Fearon did not hear from the patient for six weeks, but she then sent for him. Her state had suddenly grown worse, and her pain was now intolerable. Her first surgeon had recommended her to go to yet another surgeon, who prescribed her salivation (mercury). According to Fearon, it was expressly salivation that had made her condition worse; he was now able to persuade her to have an operation, which went well.[106]

From the case studies presented throughout, we see that it was the patient who made all decisions as to her treatment: it was only in the very last stage of the disease that the surgeon had to refuse to operate on ethical grounds. Until the end of the eighteenth century it was prohibited on ethical grounds to carry out operations on patients who were dying. The above patient referred to by Duncan finally decided not only not to have her breast removed, but also not to be tested by electricity; she even 'gave up attendance at the Dispensary, to try the effects of gentle dressings'.[107] As we see, women's agency, their will to shop around for a cure, penetrated all social strata.[108]

After hearing an unpleasant verdict, Mrs A. sought other opinions. Even though others suggested the same, she refused to follow their recommendations. Eventually she found satisfactory help from what Ewart considered a country quack:

> In May 1791, she discovered a hard knob in her left breast, about the size of a marble. Finding it increase, she had a consultation of a physician and two surgeons about three months afterwards, all of whom advised her to have it cut out. The knob was

then as large as a pigeon's egg. Dreading an operation by the knife, she applied to the country quack, who in August 1791 put a caustic to it, which kept open for three months.[109]

Elizabeth Robinson, who kept a coal-shed in Bermondsey Street, London, suffered greatly from a schirrous tumour in her breast, and was admitted to the Surrey Dispensary in April 1784, where she became Henry Fearon's patient. It is possible that she had already consulted others, since she had been told her breast was cancerous. Fearon put her on a large dose of hemlock, but she left his care in two months, having in her own opinion not received enough help from his prescriptions. She disappeared from his sight for two months. When she returned, she told him that she had gone to the Westminster Infirmary to be treated by Mr Justamond, but had not found his treatments satisfactory either, for which reason she was now returning. Fearon put her on a diet consisting of milk and vegetables, and ordered her 'four leeches to be applied every second day'. Through this regimen she lost much blood, and was considered by a friend to have become consumptive, but she regained her health and was cured.[110] Undoubtedly she was happy with the outcome of her shopping for a cure.

In desperation, Jane Brown similarly tried as many treatments as possible from Fearon, who wrote that '[s]he had taken a great many medicines, under the care and direction of some of the faculty, and likewise had recourse to quacks, and had taken various specific nostrums, but all to no purpose'. Tired of testing different treatments she finally decided to have a surgical operation, and it was successful.[111] Of another of his patients trying to find any relief, from doctors and quacks, Feraon snorted that 'notwithstanding every remedy and application that could be thought of, had been tried by regular and eminent practitioners, as well as by itinerant pretenders'.[112] These patients were clearly determined.

One of the most tenuous women I have come across was Mrs Tuckwell, who lived near Woodstock in the mid-eighteenth century. She first consulted two surgeons, the first of whom dressed her wound for half a year. Later she went to Oxford to consult an eminent surgeon, who said that the knife was needed. She refused the scalpel and went to London to see Richard Guy; but before then she had already made the decision to go to France to see surgeons there if the London surgeons all recommended a mastectomy.[113] As in Mrs Tuckwell's case, much of this shopping around was done in avoidance of the knife. The wife of a London City clergyman suffered from a horrid ulcer in her breast, which according to her doctor, Wiseman, had developed because she had not listened to his early advice. She died of her condition, and her fate made Wiseman note: 'She passed under the endeavours of many eminent Physicians and Chirurgeons of the City, but died miserably.'[114] The patient looked in many directions for a cure. The tone of the surgeon or physician in these situations is often condemnatory: had the patient come to me first, she might have been saved. In published books this message is partly included to lure more patients to the practitioner; but for us of course they also speak of the patient's process in searching for a cure.

From the patient's point of view, there were severe deterrents speaking against many of the proposed cures, amputation of the breast being the greatest woe: the operation itself caused great fear, it was life-threatening and could offer only little hope of a complete cure. But any hope was vital, and surgery offered some – at least the hope of a few more months of life. This was why, especially from the eighteenth century onwards, surgeons who otherwise might have deemed a case incurable and hopeless suggested that their patient have the diseased breast removed. Thus Mrs Cockran, aged forty-four, a patient of Rowley's, had been advised by 'an eminent hospital surgeon ... to have her breast cut off' even though the surgeon had told her that the disease was 'impossible to cure'. Mrs Cockran chose, according to Rowley, not to be cut, and sought another opinion; if we can believe Rowley, she was cured by his medications, and was still alive more than six years later.[115] She probably thought that it was her stubbornness, her keeping her own mind, that saved her breast.

Barbara Duden and Mary Fissell have reflected on the blurred and permeable boundaries of the vocabularies used by both doctors and patients: the language of diagnosis is built on both their vocabularies. The patient's story is interwoven in the physician's or surgeon's diagnosis. What was said to the patient was probably quite well understood by her, and what she said of her condition contributed to the medical professional's account of it.[116] This further confirms the notion that not only can the patient's experience be read to some extent in the physician's account, but it also speaks of the important and expected agency of the patient.

Mrs Jennings from Bedfordshire[117] speaks loudly in her surgeon Samuel Young's report. Young provided her account in his book with quotation marks, and explained that this was her own account. He had quite likely modified it, but Young put so much effort into showing he was reporting the patient's own narrative that it is credible to believe that we can hear Mrs Jenning's words. Young of course would have had the legitimate choice of using his own words. Clearly, the patient's own account was greatly valued and its authenticity was given importance. Mrs Jennings may first have consulted the physician or apothecary several months after she had noticed a lump in her breast, since she mentions that the lump had started to grow in the spring of 1810, a few months after she had first noticed it. In the summer, leeches were applied to her breast in order to at least ease the pain the lump was now causing.[118] Mrs Jennings does not mention what happened between then and 1811, when she consulted a Mr Cooper (this could be the famous surgeon); he ordered leeches to be applied regularly. She made a note of the situation, and remarked that leeches were not entirely suitable: they 'appeared to occasion a contraction of the parts affected. After some months the drawn parts (under the nipple) began to ooze, and a few large red pimples appeared near the middle.'[119] In 1812, she said, she went to see Mr Cooper again. She seems to have led that consultation: she told Mr Cooper from the first that she would not have her breast operated: 'In 1812, I again shewed it to Mr. Cooper, when upon saying I should not like to undergo an operation, as the arms appeared to be affected: he answered, it is very fortunate when the patient and surgeon agree.'[120] Perhaps Mr Cooper agreed with Mrs Jennings, or perhaps he played down her troubles to save her from the emotional turmoil which a verdict of incurable cancer would bring.

In the autumn of 1812 the red pimples of Mrs Jennings's breast began to ulcerate. As she did not mention consulting anyone at this stage, it is possible that she medicated herself with a prescription given by Mr Cooper or with some medications of her own. Her breast continued in an ulcerated state, and was painful. In fact, her other breast had '[become] afflicted' as well, in a similar manner, but was more painful than the first one.[121] Her next consultation (or at least the next one she mentions) was in the summer of 1814, when she saw 'another surgeon in Town'. This surgeon is likely to have diagnosed her ulcerated breasts as cancerous, as he gave her a grim verdict:

> In the summer of 1814, I shewed it to another surgeon in Town, who said *nothing* could be done; but added, when it was in great pain, I might put scraped carrot to the sores; and upon my saying, it never had been in much pain, he answered, perhaps not; but I must expect the pain to be extremely violent.[122]

Cancer in the final stages was considered most torturous, and the doctor's prognosis suggested cancer. Without doubt, Mrs Jennings understood perfectly what it meant that '*nothing* could be done'. By now she had lived with her lumps and ulcerations for five years. Towards the end of her account, we can hear desperation:

> In this state, I have remained with this only consolation in my mind, that some fever might release me; or that the bleeding from my breast might carry me off, before the threatened and multiplied horrors of the complaint overtook me.[123]

Mrs Jennings did not look forward to dying from the 'multiplied horrors' of breast cancer; she wanted to leave this world before the pain overtook her. She made it clear that she did not want to lay herself down on the altar of noble suffering; instead, she wanted to leave her body before it crumbled around her. Yet despite this she had not given up all hope, and continued to seek help. In December 1814 she turned to Samuel Young, who at the time had several breast cancer patients under his care. She first consulted him in Harlington, on Tuesday, 6 December. His first medical attendance upon her took place in Bedford ten days later.[124] There was still hope for her: she was still alive and according to Samuel Young doing very well, in June 1815.[125] Mrs Jennings, and the other women discussed above, show that eighteenth-century women were in control of their choice of practitioners and courses of treatments. Most were willing to try almost anything to find a cure or at least relief, and they were active in medicating themselves.

It was not always the patient who waited before making the decision to operate. It was apparently customary for surgeons and physicians to try other means before resorting to the knife. I argue that, in general, the knife was the last resort for them too, and was commonly used only when everything else failed.[126]

The time spent considering whether or not to operate was an issue which grew in importance during the long eighteenth century. Increasingly, surgery was seen as an important option in cancer treatments. But this by no means meant that surgery in practice became the first choice for most patients. Thus when at the end of the century James Latta urged that all cancerous breasts be amputated more or less immediately, he had to note that it was dangerous for the patient or the surgeon to delay because of timidity or negligence.[127] It was still common to refuse surgery at an early stage. This further argues for the great difficulty in resorting to the knife, on the part of both the surgeon and the patient. A mastectomy was so dangerous and horrendous for the patient that surgeons too found them difficult to initiate. Exactly how demanding this operation was is revealed by Latta, who elaborated upon why an advanced case should never be operated on:

> The patient's health and strength being already much impaired by the long continuance of the disease, she must undoubtedly be very little able to bear the additional pain and weakness of one of the most formidable operations which can be performed on the human body. That the amputation of a cancerous breast is a very terrible operation, even when performed in the very best manner, cannot be denied; how much worse then must it be when an hour, or perhaps more, is taken up with it, instead of twenty minutes, which ought only to be employed.[128]

Latta notes that mastectomy was 'one of the most formidable operations', 'a very terrible operation'; as though to corroborate this horribleness, he repeats his view later on.[129]

Latta argued for an early operation precisely because later it would become even more demanding and dangerous, if not altogether impossible. It was already a sixteenth-century maxim to note that when a cancer advances 'there followe more cruell tormentes, and the strength decaying by little and little, at the last the whole bodye languisheth and consumeth'.[130] It was this torment that many well-meant popular medical books appealed to in trying to frighten possible patients into having the operation. No doubt surgeons and physicians in their practices described these torments to the patients. Thus Mansey addressed his lay readers with a quotation from a specialist, Mr Parkinson:

> considering that it is highly preferable to undergo a few moments pain, and obtain relief to your mind, than to suffer the gradual increase of a disease which must become

daily more painful, and at last *must terminate in death.* – Be assured' continues he, 'that for this disease there is *no remedy known*'.[131]

The emphases above are original, and lend a very gloomy feel to the page.

Parkinson wrote in his *Medical Admonitions* that in the early stage of the disease, when the tumour was but a small kernel, the operation was 'comparatively trivial'.[132] He further tried to persuade his readers that the fear of the operation arose not only from the fear of pain but from the mental images induced by the horrible situation:

> The assemblage of the surgeons, the preparation of instruments, and many other circumstances, the enumeration of which would be opposite to the present purpose, are all represented in a colouring so *sombre*, and with touches so masterly and impressive, that the mind is filled with the utmost horror at the picture the imagination has drawn.[133]

Thus the patient could no longer reason herself into having the operation at a safe stage, but would refuse it. She had become what Parkinson termed 'the slave of terror': '[r]eason has no longer power to exert its influence; and the unfortunate sufferer, thus becoming the slave of terror, attempts not to argue and combat with the host of terrific spectres which fancy is constantly placing before the eyes'.[134] Everyday proof of this was that patients often agreed to the use of a caustic, even though its painfulness was known to be both dreadful and long-lasting.[135] Reason should say, in Parkinson's view, that it was much more sensible to suffer a few minutes' pain, even though it was 'the most excruciating pain', in order to 'procure an entire liberation from misery and despondence'.[136] And in fact many did so, and accepted surgery. They were not necessarily fearless; but they evidently put their fear aside and decided to take a chance.

On Those who Resorted to the Knife

As we have seen, patients tended not to consult surgeons in the early stages of their cancer. This meant that the actual operation typically took place after a long illness.[137] A highly typical case would be something like that of a forty-year-old woman, who finally chose to have an operation after having her tumour for seven years. It had started growing two years before she had the breast removed. In her case, too, the reason for the removal of the breast was the pain suffered. Clearly the tumour had grown a bit before there was considerable pain; it was when the pain became unbearable that she requested a surgical operation.[138]

This was the last resort: surgery was not only dangerous but guaranteed nothing and involved the risk of death. No ethical surgeon could promise a good outcome. Robert Mustow advised his young colleagues not to promise the patient too much, but that what one promised, one had to carry out well: 'perfourme faithfully what thou promise'.[139] In practice this would often have meant difficult and careful balancing between motivating the patient into having the operation and being realistic – which could hardly be anything but a pessimistic outlook.

Importantly, the surgeon was not to promise an absolute cure. Mustow motivates this reservation on several grounds. He notes that the patient's fate is not in the surgeon's hands alone, but is always based on four different factors: first, the determination of God; secondly, the 'skill & industrie of the Author', meaning the surgeon; thirdly, the art of the apothecary; and lastly, the obedience of the patient.[140] The patient was always responsible for her course of treatments.

In 1784 Jane T. suffered from a lemon-sized tumour in her right breast. The tumour had grown for several years, increasing not only in size but also in painfulness. Lately her pains had become quite severe. When she consulted a surgeon she was already prepared to have her breast operated upon. She rode several miles to see the surgeon Nooth, and when he suggested the necessity of an operation, 'she eagerly desired' that it be carried out 'on the following morning'.[141] When she had made up her mind, Jane T. clearly wanted to have it over and done with.

Jane T.'s swift decision would have pleased many proponents of surgery. As we have seen, speed was considered extremely important – even if in practice it often meant speed after first waiting for months or even years. It goes without saying that in the eighteenth century a cancer could not be identified before the tumour was large enough to be felt. Richard Guy, who himself preferred not to use the knife on cancers, thought that it was extremely important that – however reluctant the patient and however awful the operation – if it were to be done, it was better done as soon as possible. And indeed, he notes,

> it is a melancholy Sentence when Necessity obliges us to acquaint a Patient, (advanced to the utmost State of Misery) That there can be Nothing done, i.e. No Hopes of a Cure but in Death, as at that Time, most of those unhappy Persons would submit to any Thing, upon the least Prospect of a Recovery, when it is too late.[142]

Such was the case of Miss J— M—, whose cancer advanced rapidly. She had first hurt her breast in November 1761, and experienced pain for a few days afterwards. In March 1762 the cancer grew fast, and made her sufficiently concerned about the condition of her breast to seek help; she was treated for ten months with hemlock and other remedies. These treatments made no improvement, and the surgeon, Mr Hill, considered her case hopeless, saying so to her and her friends. Miss J— M— was not surprised to hear this, as she 'resolutely replied: "I believe so; but the pain is so unsupportable, that you must proceed to the operation, though I should die among your hands".[143] Again, it was the unbearable pain that made her welcome a mastectomy, even though the operation itself promised but to put an end to the pain caused by the tumour.

Similar fortitude can be found in a forty-four-year-old woman who requested
an amputation; she was suffering from horrible pains and from a stench from her
ulcerated breast, and was considered by her physicians so weak that 'the bare
mention of amputation would kill her'.[144] Because of her weak condition she was
not operated on, but was treated with hemlock. In February 1770 she finally
succumbed to a horrible fit.[145]

As already noted, even when an operation was opted for, the time period
elapsed from the first worrying signs was often considerable. Take Mrs B, who
was operated on when she was forty-six or forty-seven years old. She had received
a hurt on her breast twenty-four years earlier, and had suffered all those years
from some pains and a swelling. Over time, these had slowly increased.[146] An
amputation was never an easy solution, but as this case among other shows, in
most cases it was probably postponed until it was deemed the only way to save or
prolong the patient's life. Naturally each case was different: some tumours grew
fast, some slowly, and according to contemporary theories of cancer there were
different ways to meet the danger. Some proposed a passive approach, to wait
and see and to avoid aggravating the 'evil'. Some thought it was best to remove a
small tumour; but it was probably difficult for the patient to submit to an operation at this early a stage, before they could actually see the danger. Of course
there were exceptions to this rule as well. Mary Woodward, only sixteen years
old, first noticed the trouble in her breast around Michaelmas when part of it
became hard and swollen. In June she came from the country to London to be
operated on at St George's Hospital. At this point the swelling was the size of a
large fist.[147] It was probably this aggressive progression of the disease that was the
key to her decision to have her breast operated on.

The best-known of all women to have a mastectomy before the invention of
anaesthesia, Fanny Burney (Frances D'Arblay), was also quite typical. Madame
D'Arblay would probably not like to be described as 'average', but that is what
she was, in terms of her age, the long history of her illness, and the fact that she
survived her ordeal. What makes her case different from the others is her unique
account of her mastectomy, carried out in 1811, which she wrote for her sister
Esther.[148] The letter was started some time in the spring of 1812 – the first sheet
was dated 22 March, and it was completed in June.[149]

As I have said, Burney's report of her experience is unique. To my knowledge, there is no other equally detailed and extensive autobiographical account
of a mastectomy. Other patients, even if they survived, chose to remain silent,
were unable to write about their experience at all or did not even consider doing
so. Accounts may also have been lost. We know from Fanny Burney's account
that writing after a breast amputation was physically difficult and painful, especially when part of the breast muscle was removed. Even though her medical
care ended in the spring of 1812,[150] she was still in pain that summer: she wrote

to her husband that he should not worry about her writing, since she only used her wrist, not her shoulder muscles. As was the practice in early radical mastectomies, her breast muscle was at least partly removed, which gave her trouble. She noted that she had developed a new technique for writing: 'I have found a new way, upon a piece of board, of planting my paper that is somewhat less fatiguing.'[151] Fanny Burney analysed how difficult it was for her mentally to go through the operation again in writing:

> My dearest Esther, not for days, not for Weeks, but for Months I could not speak of this terrible business without nearly again going through it! I could not *think* of it with impunity. I was sick, I was disordered by a single question – even now, 9 months after it is over, I have a head ache from going on with the account! & this miserable account, which I began 3 Months ago, at least, I dare not revise, nor read, the recollection is still so painful.[152]

Her recollections were physically painful, giving her a headache and making her feel nauseous nine months after her operation. But more than her writing, I want to discuss Fanny Burney's mastectomy and the way she experienced it.[153] We should begin with her first sense of horror. It is significant that she remembered growing anxious about her state only when she had been visited by Monsieur Dubois, who could be considered a great authority. He was an M.D. and professor of surgery, and the Empress's *accoucheur*, man-midwife.[154] Before that she had felt no fear, but noted that it was her husband who worried, urging her to consult the surgeon. Monsieur Dubois prescribed her medicines to take for a month, and then met privately with Monsieur D'Arblay behind closed doors – significantly, the doors were closed to Mme D'Arblay herself. This negotiation was carried out without her in order to keep her spirits up, but her husband's grave face gave the verdict away. His looks were shocking to her. 'The bitterest woe', a euphemism for cancer, was legible on his face, and she knew without his saying so that she would need a surgical operation.[155]

Burney seems to have known beforehand what her options would be, and known before seeing Monsieur Dubois that having to submit to an operation would be the worst possible alternative. The matter had been discussed, and put aside, for months. On hearing the verdict, however, Burney remembered being more shocked than frightened:

> I had not, therefore, much difficulty in telling myself what he endeavoured not to tell me – that a small operation would be necessary to avert evil consequences! – Ah, my dearest Esther, for this I felt no courage – my dread & repugnance, from a thousand reasons *besides* the pain, almost shook all my faculties, &, for some time, I was rather confounded & stupified [*sic*] than affrighted.[156]

It was perhaps the shock and fear of the operation that Burney thought worsened her condition. She wrote that her all symptoms now grew worse and more serious. Her fear of the operation was in her own words 'insuperable'.[157] Because of this, Monsieur Dubois was replaced by Dominique-Jean Larrey, who had previously cured one woman with the same condition, but had actually worked as an army surgeon (thus he would have had great skill with the scalpel and extensive experience in amputations). Despite his profession, Larrey was not a knife-happy man but intended to save Burney from the feared operation; some hope resurfaced when his prescriptions made her better, even though the pains were still strong.[158] Larrey's hope of curing her without surgery was seconded to Burney's delight by Monsieur Ribes (whom she called Ribe). In all happiness, it was declared that Dubois had been wrong.[159]

But Burney's great improvement ceased and she took a turn for the worse. She received very bad news: her beloved Princess Amelia and her dear Mr Lock had both died. She believed that these adverse circumstances brought on the aggravation of her cancer.[160] Her decline seems to have been rapid: when Larrey came to see her after the last of her sad news, she was already in a bad state, and they had to give up all hope of dissolving the tumour by outward means alone.[161] It was decided by a council of three men – Larrey, Ribes and a physician named Moreau – that an operation was after all required. Burney resisted: she wrote that her 'poor breast' was not discoloured, nor was it much larger than 'its healthy neighbour'. Her choice of words is interesting, in that she personified and perhaps distanced her breasts: they were like friends that she discussed from a distance. She admitted the 'evil', as she called the growth in her breast, was to some extent frightening: 'Yet I felt the evil to be so deep, so deep, that I often thought if it could not be dissolved, it could only with life be extirpated.'[162] Here I read a candid confession of her having feared death: not, however, fear of death by cancer but by the operation. Throughout, she seems to have feared the operation more than the cancer itself, but this may be explained by the fact that she survived the operation: now that her disease was conquered, she felt that the operation itself had been the greatest hazard.

When Monsieur Dubois was again brought in to be consulted, and all four men agreed that an operation was necessary to save her life,[163] despite her terrible fear of the operation, Burney submitted. The language she uses in her letter is dramatic: she writes that she 'saw all hope was over', and that Larrey 'pronounced my doom'. She realized there was no way of escaping what she saw as the worst possible fate, and agreed to the operation. The surgeons were left to decide the date.[164]

Pain and much suffering was predicted for her: 'Vous Souffrirez – vous souffrirez *beaucoup*!', she was told.[165] At this point Burney's main concern was to make sure that her husband and son were not informed as to the date or the exact time of the operation. In fact, the surgeons decided that they would not tell Burney herself about these either; instead, she heard that she would be informed of the operation four hours beforehand, so that she could prepare herself. Thus she spent many long days in dreadful expectation. Dramatically as ever, she noted that those days were full of 'hourly expectation of a summons to execution'.[166] She does not seem to have used this kind of imagery simply for the sake of a dramatic effect, but because this was how she remembered the situation. Naturally, she feared that she might die during the operation: the operation could in fact easily have been her 'execution'.

In the morning of 30 September 1811, the feared letter was delivered to Madame D'Arblay. She was informed that Larrey would arrive with his assistants at ten o'clock. Burney replied saying she would not be ready before one o'clock, and hurried to ensure that her husband was away when the operation took place. Her sixteen-year-old son was informed, however, and was sent, crying, to bluff his father. Fanny Burney made herself busy preparing her apartment, from which her husband was now 'banished', to the operation and to her convalescence.[167] She managed to keep herself perfectly busy until one o'clock, when the operation was set to begin. This calmed her nerves. A terrible setback followed when Mr Dubois sent word that he could not attend until three o'clock. Burney's depiction of the two hours of waiting is gripping:

> I strolled to the Sallon – I saw it fitted with preparations, & I recoiled – But I soon returned; to what effect disguise from myself what I must so soon know? – yet the sight of the immense quantity of bandages, compresses, sponges, Lint – – Made me a little sick: – I walked backwards & forwards till I quieted all emotion, & became, by degrees, nearly stupid – torpid, without sentiment or consciousness; – & thus I remained till the Clock struck three.[168]

Remarkably however, Burney recovered her 'spirit of exertion' and wrote letters to her husband and son 'in case of a fatal result'. When she was finished, she heard the noises of four cabriolets coming to a stop in front of the house.[169] The sense of doom multiplies at this point of the account: the carriages stopped one by one, and her room was entered by Dr Moreau. He came, according to her, to see if she was alive, and gave her the wine cordial.[170]

The sense of doom in Burney's memoir changed to a sense of being intruded upon by seven men, when her five doctors and their two assistants, all dressed in black, entered her room without prior notice. She was 'awakened from any stupor', and felt indignation: 'Why so many? & without leave?'[171] She was alarmed by the rash nature of the procedure, and was further offended when Dr Dubois ordered that the operation be performed on a bed rather than on a chair, as they had agreed earlier. Burney remembered being unable to utter a word. To her horror, two old mattresses and old sheets – apparently in order to save new ones from being ruined with blood – were ordered for her. This was too much; she notes that she 'began to tremble violently, more with distaste & horror of the preparations even than of the pain'.[172] Her shock at being operated upon in a recumbent position probably speaks of the horizontal position being demeaning; lying down, she probably felt more violently assaulted. In a sitting position she would have been able to maintain some authority.

Next, Burney was told to get on the bed, and to remove her robe. She put up some resistance, but admitted that while she was not entirely aware of the dangers of the operation, she knew that however dangerous, inconvenient and threatening it might be, she had to go through with it in order to save her life.[173] Thus she climbed onto the bed, lay down, and had her face covered with a cambric handkerchief. It was so transparent that she could see the horrors of the operation through it.[174] Then, finally, she submitted, closed her eyes and was ready to meet her fate; she relinquished 'all watching, all resistance, all interference, & sadly resolute to be wholly resigned'.[175]

The next twenty minutes,[176] which was the duration of the operation, were horrible, and the following months, filled with post-operational pain, were an ordeal. As though to prove this, she told her sister that it took months before she was able to talk about her ordeal without having to relive the pain; she could 'not *think* of it with impunity'.[177] These afterthoughts caused both mental and physical pain; added to which was undoubtedly the physical pain caused by her wound, her mutilated chest.

Like Fanny Burney, countless women survived lumpectomies and mastectomies, which certainly gave encouragement to those who followed in their footsteps. Astonishing to our present-day sensibilities, there were even women who considered the benefits of the operation so great that they preferred to go through the experience again when their disease recurred. Some women were operated on twice or even several times. There are also some hints as to the possibility that some women had both breasts removed. There were hardly many of these; surgeons were supposed to categorically refuse to operate on cases that were pronounced incurable, and recurring cancers were considered hopeless and beyond the help of the knife.[178] Thus, for example, William Rowley's patients included a couple of women who had had an operation, but in whose case he refused to operate on the other breast because he considered recurring cases hopeless.[179]

Not all doctors chose this line, however. The diary of Richard Kay, a country physician and surgeon, reveals a different attitude.[180] He went to extremes to help a patient, Mrs Driver.[181] Mrs Driver had decided that her diseased breast had to be amputated. Kay operated on it in December 1748. His entry for 22 December 1748 notes that after taking care of some household things, he and his father (also a practitioner) went to Mr Driver's house at Crowshaw-Booth. This was of course 'according to Apointment'. He writes: 'with the Assistance of my Father I took off Mrs. Driver's right Breast that was Cancerous, the Cancer weighed near 3 Pound Weight'.[182] The tumour was quite large, and as always there was a risk of post-operation bleeding; this was the reason why Kay stayed at the Drivers' house for two nights, and then left Mrs Driver 'in good Order'.[183] For our purposes, Kay's diary does not yield much concerning his patient, who remains rather faceless, but what does become clear is that Kay was a good surgeon: he visited his patient the following day, which was Christmas Day. The published diary does not mention a visit on Boxing Day, but he went there again on 27 and 29 December.[184] These visits were made to change her dressings, as he mentions explicitly in his entry of 10 January 1748/9. On 10 January Mrs Driver is first given a voice, but it is on his behalf: Kay mentions that she had heard of his accident on his horse,[185] and they talked about the wonder of him being unhurt. His great piety is reflected in what he recollects then saying:

> I answered, that I believed we both fared better for the Prayers and good Wishes of our Friends; that as she had been wonderfully preserved and supported in her Afflic-tion, so Providence might see God to shew an Instance wherein he wou'd preserve and support me tho' in imminent Danger. Lord, I believe in Providence, and have more than common Dependance upon it; strengthen and increase my Faith and Trust, and preserve me both in Body and Soul.[186]

Mrs Driver recovered well from the operation, and had been 'hearty' for several months before she unfortunately returns to Kay's professional life. His entry on 7 June 1749 is dramatic, and I quote it in full:

> This Day in the Morning I was employed in some Domestick Affairs, in the After-noon I visited Mrs. Driver at Crowshaw-Booth the person whose Cancerous Breast I took off twenty second Day of last December, the Wound cured, and she had been hearty some Months; last Saturday she came here to Baldingstone to shew us a Knot she had discovered that Morning about an Inch and a half below the old Wound upon the Forepart of her Ribs, which growing so fast upon the Sunday, Monday, &c. Mrs. Driver came here for us she being determined to undergo a second Amputation, upon dissecting the Knot I soon found I had more Work to do than was expected as there appeared other Kernalls closely joyned together which lay down to the Abdo-men and the Compass of six or seven Inches square, in some Parts I took off the Skin, in others dissected them from under the Skin, so that from below where her Breast formerly was down her Ribs to her Belly I dissected from her at a moderate Computa-tion five hundred different distinct Schirrous Knots or young Cancers; she was sick and very poorly after the Operation. I lodge at Mrs. Driver's. Lord, May we have hope towards God and may this support and comfort us under the different Occurrences in Life, yea under the severest Afflictions and Death itself.[187]

In the eyes of her contemporaries, as well as our own, Mrs Driver must have been a courageous woman. She was an agent in her own life, and took immediate action when she noticed the 'Knot'. That very day she had gone to Baldingstone to show it to Kay, and we have to believe Kay was not lying when he noted that she was 'determined to undergo a second Amputation'. I tend to read Kay's last sentence in the cited entry to indicate that he believed Mrs Driver had only little hope. His simple prayers, added as a reflection on the day, often referred to his cases.

Kay respected her demand to be operated on again and removed hundreds of kernels from her chest, even though he knew the cancer was spreading unstoppably. This, however, was not enough. Mrs Driver had a third operation on 8 July. This time tumours were removed from her neck and shoulder. Her state was then 'afflicted', but the operation went well. Kay seems to have been certain that her end was near. He closes this entry as follows: 'Lord, Prepare us for Death and for a happy and glorious Eternity'.[188] A fourth operation took place on 14 August, at which time Kay removed cancers in the area between her armpit and shoulder.[189] He visited her again on 4 September, although mentions nothing of the purpose of his visit,[190] but on 25 and 30 September he again removed more tumours. On 25 September three relatively large tumours of the size of eggs were removed, and on 30 September he removed several from the old wound.[191] On 5 October he again mentions having operated on her,[192] and visited her at least on 2 January, 1749/50. The last entry referring to her is from 20 February, the date of her funeral. She had probably been released from her great ordeal the previous day.[193]

Mrs Driver had a kindred spirit in forty-year-old Elizabeth Auger, who had a very aggressive cancer. The nature of the cancer is probably why she was eager to undergo surgery almost at the first onset of the cancer, and she too had more than one operation. Auger was admitted to the Surrey Infirmary only three weeks after the first onset of her symptoms. Her state was poorly: her right breast was enlarged, her 'countenance was pale and sickly, she was subject to indigestion, and frequent nausea', and there were frequent darting and pricking pains in her breast. Moreover, there were diseased glands everywhere in the breast, as well as in the axilla.[194] I have argued that women did not usually resort to the knife at the first instance, but here the case seems to be the very opposite. Indeed, only three weeks' illness brought her to the certainty that an operation was necessary. She wanted to have an operation because 'the disease had increased so rapidly'. According to her surgeon Fearon, she 'intreated' him 'in the most earnest manner to perform the operation, and give her a chance for her life'.[195] It is very likely that Auger was eager to have an operation because she had been given hope from meeting two of Fearon's patients whom he had cured with his knife.[196]

Fearon considered Auger's disease so dangerous and so far gone that he thought 'that it must end fatally' – or so he later wanted his readers to believe. I am inclined to believe his words. He gained nothing from this frankness, and as it was not customary to operate on such advanced cases he might actually have been inviting the disapproval of many of his colleagues. He agreed to operate on Auger, and was appalled at how widely the disease had spread: he was 'very much alarmed', as he had to remove 'an incredible number' of knots.[197] Auger healed well, and for two months was in perfect health. According to Fearon, she 'thought herself very fortunate'. But it was not to last: the disease returned. With her breast almost as large as before the operation, she returned to Fearon. She was now given hemlock, but it did not ease her situation, and he pronounced her case hopeless. But Auger was by no means willing to give up quite yet: she wanted another operation:

> I feared it would not be in my power to remove the whole diseased mass, she had but little reason to expect any benefit from having the operation repeated ... as she suffered such constant and severe pain, she was resolved to undergo the operation a second time.[198]

Again, Fearon complied. All the cancerous growth in her breast and axilla was removed, and she again soon healed. For three months her happiness must have been great, as she enjoyed good health. But once more the disease returned, 'and in a short time, shot out in different directions to a great size, large lumps or pieces frequently mortifying and sloughing away with the poultices that were then applied'. For five more months she lived in great suffering. Opium no longer helped, and she could neither sleep nor find ease from the pain. This was the end of her fierce fight against death: 'thus worn out with want of rest, incessant pain, and hectic fever, she died'.[199] Auger, from Wandsworth Road, indeed fought for her life, and even against the advice of her surgeon was willing to go though the horrible operation twice. She was the epitome of female agency.

Mrs S. was from Coventry, and at the time when she saw her chosen surgeon, Mr Wilmer, on 12 March 1772, she was suffering from a ten-month-old schirrus tumour in her right breast. It was not attached to any tissues, and thus promised a cure with the knife. She was operated on two days after she first saw Wilmer. Unfortunately, in four months time there appeared another tumour near her axilla, which grew daily, and was painful. She was now treated with a large dose of hemlock, and two London surgeons, Mr Sharp and Mr Harrold, were consulted. They suggested another operation. Since the disease had advanced so rapidly and the danger of adhesion was present, she agreed, and was operated on again on 2 November 1772. In fact, the tumour had already adhered to the edge of the pectoral muscle, part of which was now removed. This time the wound was not closed at the first incision, but was kept open. Nothing, however, helped. Her cancer spread at an alarming rate, and when the ulcer 'corroded some large branches of the artery', she died.[200]

Many patients were extremely obstinate and insisted on an operation even when it was strictly against the advice of the surgeons they consulted. A prime example is the case of a feisty young woman with hard glands in her breast. She had consulted several experts, and had come to Wiseman to be operated on immediately. She insisted on an instant lumpectomy, but Wiseman refused. He wanted to prepare her body first, to purge and bleed her and have her humours 'better disposed'. During the weeks this took, she consulted someone else, and again insisted that the glands be removed. Wiseman once again refused; he considered the glands too deep for extirpation to be an option, and that the whole breast would have to be removed. This is not what she wanted, and she had the glands removed by another surgeon only a few days after that consultation. The breast, unfortunately, grew cancerous, as Wiseman had predicted, and the surgeon had to remove the whole breast in another operation. She later came to see him with an ulcerated breast, the ulcer 'deep and wide into the pectoral Muscle and Parts about, and fixed to the Ribs'. Wiseman could no longer do anything but ease her pains. As he wrote, he learned from this case that one should not cut off breasts that grew cancerous from inward causes.[201]

Similarly obstinate and determined was a fifty-year-old woman who had schirrous glands in her breast and impatiently wanted them removed. Her surgeon was the same Wiseman, and he refused to comply in her case as well. She refused to settle down and die, and turned to 'empyricks', but unfortunately things turned worse. Wiseman tells us that he had to mend the damage. She had bled nearly to death, and he could hardly stop her bleeding. He noted that her tumour was 'a meer fungus', and not immediately dangerous. She recovered from her ordeal, even though there was another lump in her armpit, which was treated. About a year later a friend of hers, Mrs R., 'who laboured of a Cancer in her Breast', had a mountebank cut off her breast. She was thus cured, our patient said, and demanded once again that Wiseman cut off her breast. He once more refused; he thought he had talked her out of her idea, and left her to her own devices. She had decided otherwise, however: she sent for an empiric, and was applied escharotics. 'She bled to death in few days', he wrote, and added that she had sent for him in this situation, but that he had been out of London, and she had died before he arrived. He concludes by acknowledging that it was the patient who made the decisions: 'If she had not been in such haste, she might have out-lived that Gentlewoman: for her Breast became cancerous, and she died in few Months after.'[202]

What emerges from the great majority of sources is the patients' agency and their given right to their bodies. These women decided for themselves. Some of them were so obstinate they were in fact quite unruly. As patients, they chose their doctors and surgeons as long as they had the financial means to do so or were accepted as non-paying patients. As patients, they sometimes astonished their physicians and surgeons by behaving in an unruly manner and against their professional advice; but this was considered acceptable, even if – when the chosen path ended in an early grave – regrettable. No one could guarantee a favourable outcome with an illness such as cancer.

4 'SO FRIGHTFUL TO THE VERY IMAGINATION':[1] PAIN, EMOTIONS AND CANCER IN THE BREAST

In early modern culture as well as in eighteenth-century thinking, fear was a dangerous emotion. It could cause illness and even kill. Because cancer in the breast was known to be one of the most horrible diseases it was also greatly feared, and contemporaries, both doctors and laymen, thought that the fear of cancer could in fact generate cancer in certain situations, especially if fear was overwhelming. Many people were in contact with patients and had intimate knowledge of the terrifying effects of advanced cancer; this knowledge would make many people extremely fearful and prone to suspect the worst if their breasts gave any worrying signs such as darting pains or lumps. I have written elsewhere on the great fears Margaret Baxter and Anna Seward had when they showed such symptoms.[2] Margaret Baxter was the wife of Richard Baxter, the puritan theologist, and he attested in his *A Breviate of the Life of Margaret* that his wife had in fact died because of her sensitive nature: by worrying about cancer she weakened her body, and eventually died, very likely believing she had cancer in the breast.[3] Anna Seward had a more positive fate, but she too was devastated by her fears of cancer. Threatening symptoms started up after she accidentally hurt her breast 'by slipping against the sharp-pointed ledge of a wainscot'. She was pained by fears and by her breast for two years, but in the end the fears luckily proved futile: the hurt in the breast did not turn cancerous. At times she had been so desperate that she wrote she envied an early grave.[4]

Fear could indeed overwhelm. In the early eighteenth century, one of Daniel Turner's patients had lumps in her breasts, and he advised her to have them safely removed so as never to be bothered with them again. The patient, a young gentlewoman, was nearly certain that she had cancer; she consulted other doctors, who prescribed a number of different medications, including the fashionable millipedes and sarsaparilla. She took these medications for three months, but saw no change in her breast. Turner then advised her to discontinue taking either medicine and to leave her breast alone: she would be well following his advice. He thought it was all the different remedies that were making her life miserable, but all for nothing: 'it was my Advice, that she might throw off her

Regimen, and live no longer physically, that is miserably, but prudently take her Food of Meats easily concocted, with agreeable Diversion, and above all, giving her Breast Liberty, to forbear handling it herself, or admitting others so to do'.[5] Following Turner's advice, the patient was soon free of trouble from the breast; she later married and had 'several children'. While the trouble her lump gave her had ceased, the tumour did not dissolve from her breast. It remained unaltered, stone-like, but caused no further harm.[6]

Nearly a century later, Jane T., a servant in the household of the Earl of Ilchester, had at the age of twenty-eight a lemon-sized tumour in her right breast. Her condition was mentioned to a lady, who was benevolent enough to recommend Jane T. to James Nooth, a surgeon popular with polite society (when his *Observations* were published in the early nineteenth century, Nooth was surgeon to the Duke of Kent). Jane T. travelled several miles on horseback to see Nooth and to hear his verdict on her tumour. She probably braced herself to face the worst, since she was not in a healthy state. Nooth notes that Jane T.'s health had suffered and was 'evidently impaired'; her menses, however, continued normally, which was a good sign. The fear of cancer had become just as dangerous to her health as the lemon-sized tumour in her breast: he notes that 'apprehensions of a cancer had much depressed her spirits'.[7] This depression of spirits alone could deprive her of her health, not to speak of the depressing force of the tumour itself. Another patient of Nooth's, a lady's maid, aged twenty-six, who had found a tumour in her breast almost three years earlier, had been consumed by the pains she had suffered for a year before consulting Nooth. 'Her health was impaired, and her spirits much depressed', he notes, not unlike the case of Jane T.; Nooth does not specify whether or not she had felt fear.[8] We can probably assume that she feared the disease, and that it was this fear that made her depressed.[9]

Nooth diagnosed Jane T.'s tumour as a schirrous one, which for him meant a benign tumour, with the potential to turn cancerous. He recommended that it be operated on – he mentions that he 'hinted the necessity of an operation'[10] – and Jane T. was ready and prepared to accept the offer. She was eager to have the lump out, and wanted to have the operation carried out right away. Nooth refused this, however, on the grounds of her fatigue from riding all the way to see him, and the operation was postponed one or two days until she had recovered from her travel.[11] The operation went well, and she recovered her health within a fortnight.[12]

Jane T.'s illness, according to Nooth, was not yet cancerous, and she was probably most relieved to recover from her operation and go on with her life. But this was not the lot of all those who suspected the worst. It goes without saying that a diagnosis of cancer changed lives. Several recurring emotions become apparent from texts describing this phase. Melancholy was a dominant passion, especially since the diagnosis brought desperate apprehensions about the nearness of death. It could also take the form of 'extreme dejection of spirits'. Anxiety too was present, and a great fear of death: 'In these Cases it often happens, that, after having been frequently disappointed in their Expectation of Relief or a Cure, the Patients are apt to fall into an extreme Dejection of Spirits, attended with a perpetual Anxiety of Mind, and the most melancholy Apprehensions of the worst Consequences.'[13]

The sufferings felt by the patient were an ethical issue for the treating doctor, and according to ethical injunctions given to surgeons, they were not to cause pain: they were to work 'safely without hurt'.[14] This of course meant that the surgeon was not to cause any excessive pain which did not arise naturally out of the operation. And the patient must not be tormented: an operation considered beyond the capabilities of the patient to endure was not to be performed. The French surgeon Pierre Dionis touched upon the mental state of the patient – and the need for the surgeon to recognize this:

> The Prognostic must necessarily be very melancholy since there is no Disease more afflicting, and which ought to strike the Patient with more Apprehension than an ulcerated Cancer; nor is there any way which fatigues the Chirurgeon more, nor gives him more Trouble, because the Disease is almost always incurable.
>
> [...]
>
> But how are you to resist the Persecutions of a poor suffering Patient, which implores your Help? Are you to abandon her to the Rigour of her Distemper, which torments her Day and Night? No, a Chirurgeon must not be so cruel: He must search out Means to cure her: And if that is not in his Power, he must a least endeavour to soften the Disease, and render it more supportable.[15]

Dionis stressed the role of the surgeon in easing the patient's anguish. He later commented that ''tis not by Words, but by Effects that we conquer and destroy this Evil'. For him, the passions of the patient were a matter of the surgeon's ethics. His comments suggest that an illness as devastating as cancer was hardly taken lightly by surgeons – in fact, an ulcerated cancer fatigued the surgeon as well. Ethically, the desperate, fearful patient was in Dionis's view in need of the best possible care, and he considered it worthwhile to operate if at all possible.

Fear of Surgery

I next discuss the fear of surgery and the operations which were needed in the course of treating the illness. This fear was naturally inextricably linked to the fears felt towards the disease itself and cannot be analysed completely separately. Apparently, however, it was fear of the surgery that had a greatest effect, especially on the surgeon's business; hence it is therefore much more prominent in my sources than fear of the disease itself. A fearful patient often decided not to have an operation, a choice which understandably many surgeons lamented. To continue with Dionis, and to illustrate this question, we can take a look at one of his case histories: the case of a Madame de Montreuil, who had long suffered from a tumour in her breast. She now heard that she had two options: an operation or death. Her mind was probably in turmoil, and she had to make a decision quickly. Dionis reported having 'told her, that the Operation seem'd more frightful before, than it was painful or insupportable afterwards; upon which, she, like all other Patients, preferring Life to the Loss of a Member, determin'd to undergo it'.[16] Madame de Montreuil feared surgery enormously, but Dionis seems to have been convincing in his effort to turn her mind to accepting it. The operation was in his opinion much less terrifying than she had anticipated, and well worth the temporary pain.

For similar reasons apparently, Henry Fearon put some effort into trying to persuade readers not to be afraid of surgical operations. There was less cause to fear them than people generally thought, while on the positive side there was the possibility of a radical cure and of prolonging one's life significantly. Fearon admitted the fear was overwhelming:

> In these complaints, though the operation be the only alternative to which the patients must have recourse in order to preserve life, yet it requires a greater degree of resolution than most of them can readily summon up, to submit to it. The certainty of very severe and acute pain during the operation, as well as of that which must naturally follow it, the fear of a great effusion of blood, the uncertainty of success, the long confinement, and, in many cases, mutilation and deformity, are difficulties of considerable magnitude, and not easily surmounted.[17]

Fearon's words confirm that the fear of the operation was more complex than merely the fear of acute pain. Fear of surgery inevitably included the fear of sudden death during or right after the operation, and the long and possibly painful convalescence. Interestingly, he realized that many patients may have feared 'mutilation and deformity' as well, and suggested that the appearance of one's body mattered in deciding whether or not to have an operation.

For those who had 'an unconquerable aversion to the knife', and they were many, (chemical) caustics should be used, Fearon thought, recommending arsenic as the best possible caustic.[18] Similarly, Richard Guy thought it better not to use the knife but to apply Plunkett's poultice:

> Let the impartial Reader consider, how far preferable my Method is to the Knife; the very Apprehension of which carries such Terrors, that few of the Unhappy, labouring under these Complaints, can, with any Degree of Constancy, support; and often rather choose to linger out a miserable Life, than to comply with the Operation. Is it not therefore some Advantage, that Relief may be had by more gentle Means? This is mentioned, as only one superior Benefit. But to this I may add, from Experience, that it is also more certain in its Consequences.[19]

Guy's arsenic-containing remedy was quite well known, and his words were intended to form the picture of a compassionate man (it is not our task to determine the degree of his sincerity); one who sought the best for his patients and was unwilling to press them into surgery. As the following eloquent quotation suggests, he considered womenfolk especially in need of considerate treatment:

> for the most resolute of Mankind rarely submit to cutting without the last Necessity, and even then with much Reluctance. Among the Tender Sex, who are more particularly subject to cancerous Complaints, their Timidity is often found to be so great, as to rather suffer them to undergo the Miseries attendant on the Disease, and almost Death itself, before they can be brought to a Compliance with it.[20]

Women were especially in need of considerate treatment because of their timid nature, which was natural to women: they were naturally inclined to seek shelter in their homes and with men. A woman was not to be bold and assertive – timidity was a feminine virtue. Fear in a creature like this was especially dangerous. Even if we consider Guy's words to be plain sales-talk – an advertisement to attract patients in a large market, and an attempt to justify his methods, claiming their superiority to those available to the knife-wielding surgeon – it is nevertheless safe to assume that fear indeed played a major role in the patient's choice of treatment. Fearon's cases show this clearly. Mrs Elizabeth Ellis from Camberwell was recommended by several doctors to have her breast cut off, but she could not bring herself to do it. According to Fearon, this was because

> she never could make up her mind to submit to so horrid and painful an operation, which in the end might not prove successful; and to use her own words, this opinion was riveted more firmly in her mind, from the sufferings of a neighbour of her's, who had undergone the operation, under the care of one of the first surgeons in town, and gave her a dreadful account of the pain of the operation, as well as the confinement and dressings for several months.[21]

As we see, a frightening example deterred Elizabeth Ellis from having the operation. Yet examples worked in the other direction as well: it was the encouraging example of a Mrs Smith, one of Fearon's patients, that persuaded Mrs Ellis to press Fearon to amputate her breast, even though by that time her case was considered too advanced and he had become reluctant. She had met this Mrs Smith, and saw that she was doing well after her operation, and Elizabeth Ellis consequently became adamant that the sufferings caused by the operation and its consequences were less than what she would suffer without one, even though she might eventually die of cancer.[22] Overcoming the fear of an operation took determination and courage; it also required reflecting upon one's life and one's aspirations – and facing one's fears of pain and death.

The effects of breast cancer, or what was thought to be breast cancer, were devastating. In his *Seventy Four Select Cases*, Dr William Rowley notes of a Mrs Allen, who had a hardness of the breast (she had consulted several eminent practitioners, but nothing improved her condition): 'the patient became exceedingly reduced, from the tortures *and* anxiety of mind; not having the least prospect of being cured, or even relieved'.[23] It seems that the fear of death and futile attempts to cure the disease both had similar effects on the mind and body; or possibly the effect was combined.

Mrs Allen's is not an isolated case within the corpus of Rowley's twenty-four case histories treating women's breast illnesses, most of them different kinds of tumours. Like Mrs Allen, Mrs Finch was, according to Rowley, greatly consumed by the fear arising from the prospect of the disease and by the treatments she had undergone under the administrations of less knowledgeable colleagues. Her breast had swollen and there were swellings in the armpit as well; with such severe problems, it is no wonder she thought she was going to die. Rowley considered her of 'a delicate constitution' and 'very nervous'. Her anxiety, and what was probably a great fear of the disease and the ensuing death, had left her very poorly indeed. In Rowley's words, 'her anxiety of mind joined with the disorder, had brought on a universal relaxation of the habit'.[24] This is very similar to the state described by Anna Seward during her ordeal. Much of this talk – such expressions as women being of a 'delicate constitution' or 'very nervous' – reflect the ways in which women were culturally perceived in general. Their culturally constructed constitution constructed women's illnesses as well.

Mrs Stout had suffered from exquisite pains, which had 'greatly emaciated and relaxed the whole habit'.[25] This relaxation of the 'whole habit', or universal relaxation, could be the result of both bodily and mental pain. It was something Rowley apparently accepted as an effect of a disease like this, and from his political point of view as an effect of poor medical care.

Long Lasting Pains

Even with their fears and tumours, women seem to have been very patient. Anne Wildman, a poor woman from the Bedford House of Industry, apparently lived with 'jaggings' – her own expression, according to her doctor – i.e. darting pains from her tumour, for two or three years before having leeches applied by a surgeon; these abated her pain, at least temporarily, after each application. Although these jaggings denied her proper rest, she seems to have been patient with her ailment; but when the tumour began to grow faster than it apparently had before, she became frightened and sprang into action. Clearly, a rapid growth in the diseased breast was an alarming sign for her. She wanted to stop the use of leeches because she thought they aggravated the tumour: 'It growed apace, and I became frightened', she explained to doctor Young when he asked her why she wanted to discontinue the leeching.[26]

In 1796 Mrs S., wife of the reverend S. S. of Bath, came to see James Nooth, senior surgeon at the Bath hospital. In his later book, Nooth notes that Mrs S.

'had long concealed a tumour in her breast',[27] but does not mention why she did so. Was she fearful? Mrs S. was thirty-eight years old, and in Nooth's judgement 'of a tender constitution and nervous temperament'.[28] Did she want to save herself from a terrifying diagnosis as long as possible? In the end she consulted Nooth, who recommended an operation. It took her a few days to make up her mind, but she agreed to it. I assume the operation was a lumpectomy, since Nooth later notes that after the operation her breast was bound up; had it been amputated, he would rather have spoken of dressing the wound.[29] Nooth remarks that she had 'declared it [the operation] infinitely less painful than she had expected'.[30]

Mrs Ball from Elsetree, Herefordshire, apparently feared a surgical operation so much that she decided she would rather let cancer kill her – a fate less immediate and seemingly, for her, more manageable to cope with. In Guy's interpretation,

> the terror of such an operation rendered her incapable of submitting to the knife. She came to town, and applied also to another eminent surgeon in Chancery-Lane, who strenuously advised her to have her breast cut off without delay, as the last and only resource left for her recovery: but still the dreadful apprehensions of such an expedient acted so powerfully upon her, that it counteracted every other consideration, and determined her to resign herself to the fatality of the disease, rather than undergo such an operation.[31]

When in fear, these women made decisions about their lives, and led them in the way that suited them best. Some feared the disease so much that they wanted to remove a tumour immediately, while for others the greatest source of fear lay in the treatments. It seems to me that many decisions were based on an intimate knowledge of someone else's (relatively) positive experience and outcome; it was comforting to know a woman who had fared well with an operation and had recovered.

For the modern woman, a mastectomy without anaesthesia seems nothing less than the source of ultimate pain and horror. Undoubtedly it was such for most early modern women as well. It is thus remarkable that many women who underwent a breast operation in early modern England seem to have thought otherwise. In 1778 Mrs A., a twenty-six-year-old married woman from Dorsetshire, had discovered a lump in her breast and had at first 'for many months disregarded it'. When the lump caused her some pain she had consulted an apothecary, who prescribed a lotion with which she might wash the breast. The tumour, however, grew and the pain increased, and she became alarmed. A 'former medical friend' attempted to destroy the tumour by caustic medicines, which torturous treatments lasted for several months. In contrast, her operation, performed in 1782 (probably a lumpectomy, since it saved much of her breast) was soon over, and after it she was able to walk to her bed. She had her arm supported by a pillow and her pains abated by an 'anodyne draught', even though, as her surgeon Nooth notes, 'she did not complain of much uneasiness'.[32]

When Nooth visited Mrs A. in the morning, she had slept well and was 'comfortably easy'. Perhaps everything really did go this well, and Nooth was not much embroidering the situation. Perhaps she indeed was happy that she had ultimately resolved to have the tumour removed; certainly she must have thought about the possibility much earlier. She had most probably agreed to cautery because she wanted to save her breast. If we are to trust Nooth's words, she was relieved to have come to him: 'She assured me, that she really experienced less pain by the operation, than she had suffered day by day after the ulcer had been treated by the caustic dressing.'[33] Mrs A. must have considered her choosing the operation a wonderful thing, since she survived her long ordeal. Fifteen years later, in 1797, Nooth adds that she was doing well. He mentions he met her then because 'she brought her youngest daughter to Bath for my advice'.[34]

Miss T., a thirty-three-year-old woman, had similarly pursued different treatments so as to deal with her illness without having to resort to the knife. When these treatments failed, she finally resolved to have an operation. Nooth writes that she 'declared the pain trifling to what her imagination had led her to expect'.[35] This does not seem overtly illogical: months of torment compared to a single though severe agony which lasted only minutes – as we recall, mastectomies rarely lasted more than twenty minutes, and lumpectomies inevitably less – was perhaps, at least for some, ultimately the easier option. Ethically bound, the surgeon had to be quick: he had to carry out the operation 'speedily without detracting tyme'[36] because he was not allowed to cause any extra pain. We must remember, however, that it is quite likely that Nooth added these assurances to his account because it fortified his message: tumours should be excised, and the short-term pain of the operation was worth suffering if one considered the benefits. Perhaps it was meant to attract more patients to his care; perhaps it was meant to show that an operation, even though most feared, was not always the worst option available.

Cancer Pain

As we have seen, many of the feelings and emotions which cancer aroused were caused by pain and the fear of pain. Now that I have discussed the fear of cancer, it is time to look at the feeling of pain or the understanding of cancer pain.[37] The fear of cancer, it seems to me, was mostly fear of the pain this disease caused in the body. Here I look at the many meanings of cancer pain and the various forms in which it manifested itself.

Anyone who feared having breast cancer or was given the diagnosis faced the fact that pain was to be expected from two sources. It was well known that the disease itself caused terrifying pain as it progressed, and for many it was painful from early on. In addition, and hardly less terrifying, the patient could expect treatments that would be horribly painful. Most treatments known to be effective in halting the progress of the disease – or curing it altogether – were known to cause immense pain. Surgical treatments – cautery and the knife – were particularly painful, to the extent that fear of this pain played an important role in the patient's choice of treatment.[38]

Nisbet thought the pain of cancers in the stomach and womb to be the worst, but nevertheless considered all cancer pain to be torture. Opium might prove ineffectual, and the pain might 'throw the patient into faintings and convulsions'.[39] Pain and cancer were inextricably linked; it was agreed that pain followed cancer.

Since the pain caused by cancer was one diagnostic indicator of the disease, recognizing the nature of the pain was of great consequence: 'A Cancer, in general, is a schirrous tumour, which, by a successive progress, becomes exquisitely painful, and attended with shootings, as it were, now and then darting; which is called dolor lancinans.'[40] The pain had a specific and recognizable nature, but in order to recognize it a certain kind of language was needed. Pains were described in certain ways, and as we saw earlier, this language often seems to have been shared by patients and practitioners. In the late eighteenth century the medical vocabulary was often specialised. In their practical diagnostics, practitioners would interpret the patient's account of pain in medical terms. The patient's *darting pain* would become the doctor's *dolor lancinans*.

Pain followed the illness; as is plain, it was usually considered to grow stronger as time passed and the patient's condition worsened.[41] A rather typical case is that of a poor woman who had a deeply ulcerated cancer, containing 'an intolerable foetid slough', and 'discharging a thin putrid ichor in great quantities'. As Burrows describes it, '[h]er disorder was attended with acute, burning, and pricking pains, which depriving her of rest, reduced her to a very emaciated state'.[42]

The stage when the tumour ulcerated was considered invariably excruciating. The process is well described in the following extract from 1670:

> Where Cancers in the Breasts are painful, there is also attending a Pulsation, or beating like a Pulse, together with a Heat more than ordinary; and where the Pains are very sharp, so as if the Part was struck with a Dart, [there] the Matter is very corrosive, and will certainly in a little time break forth in a Gleeting or some dangerous stinking Ulcer; and when they are Ulcerated, as frequently they are, from the breaking of some of the Tubercls [sic] lying under the Skin, whether the Matter that runs be much or little, the Ulcer is painful and very stinking, and not only discharge a stinking Gleety Humour, but also there thrusts forth hard and painful Lips, which in time, if not rightly managed, fixes to the Ribs (that is, if the Cancer be in the Breast or side of it) becoming, by the quick progress it makes, of a horrible and frightful appearance.[43]

According to Pierre Dionis, the source of the pain of ulceration was the flesh-eating 'serosity' of cancer matter. When the skin broke, and the ulcer was formed, 'the Pain', he wrote, was 'incomparably augmented' and would not 'allow the Patient any Relaxation'.[44] John Ball too considered the pains of ulcerated cancer the most severe:

Of all pains, that is the worst which feels to the patient like actual fire burning within the scirrhus; for then the integuments of the occult cancer are gradually distended by the increasing of its bulk, and eroded b the greater acrimony. We are therefore to endeavour, by all possible means, to prevent a cancer's becoming ulcerous. For when the skin is once broken, a dismal scene is opened, and nothing but a miserable death to be expected, the cancerous humour most greedily devouring the fleshy substance wherever it comes, and being of a caustic nature it corrodes and destroys the nerves and blood-vessels; from whence ensues a profuse loss of the vital fluid, and most commonly immoderate haemorrhages (fluxes of blood) conclude the doleful tragedy, bringing on their much desired and welcome death.[45]

That cancer was inexpressibly painful was a common notion. John Ball described its consequences as 'the severe pains and tortures that naturally attend this cruel malady'.[46]

This was consuming pain. Justamond described the effects of the pain of his patient, who had suffered for years: 'Long continuance of excruciating pain had reduced her to an extreme degree of weakness and emaciation. Her countenance was become quite livid. The disease was much advanced in its progress, both with respect to the number and condition of the sores, and the extent and size of the indurations.'[47] According to Ball, in these desperate cases death came as a relief; the 'doleful tragedy' was the painful road to death, paved by the illness. I shall return to this aspect of the illness in the concluding part of this chapter.

In London, John Burrows described the horrible experience of his patient Mary Smith, whose illness was pronounced as incurable but whom Burrows succeeded in healing, as follows:

Mary Smith opposite Mr. Rowbottom's, japanner, in Long Acre, had laboured many years under a cancer of an enormous size, during the growth of which she suffered much uneasiness. After divers applications without relief, she was advised, as the only means remaining, to have her breast taken off, but would not submit to so terrible an operation. At length she was recommended to me, in a state truly deplorable, her pains being so excruciating, as to deprive her of all rest by night and by day.[48]

The lack of rest was one grave consequence of enduring pain. We meet it so very often in these descriptions of illness that it suggests that bodily exhaustion was considered a torment in itself, and possibly served the doctor as a sign of the intensity of the patient's pain. That in turn would be an indicator of the severity of the illness, and its possible progress. Lack of sleep was also alarming because it was in itself extremely dangerous to one's health, perhaps even fatal. Sleeplessness caused by pain is an important theme in Betty Anton's case history as well.

Betty Anton was twenty-two years old, a servant, when she was admitted to the Edinburgh Infirmary by James Gregory on February 1789. He released her from the hospital on 16 March. Three days earlier Gregory took on another patient, a widow, Christie McKenzie, aged thirty-six. Both these women had undefined pains and suffered from a panoply of symptoms. They both had severe breast problems and were in great pains. Let us first take a look at Anton, the young servant. When he admitted her, Gregory recorded a brief description of her case. For the past six months her 'left Mamma has been occasionally affected with a painful distension, & externally assuming a livid hue'; this was considered a serious symptom, and often a symptom of cancer as well. What must have been extremely worrisome to Anton herself was the haemorrhage from the nipple. At the examination Gregory did not consider the breast to look 'any way diseased', but noted that fourteen months earlier there had been an ulceration, a superficial one, on the surface, joined with much discomfort in the axilla. The glands had not been enlarged, which of course was a good sign. Here too a blow to the breast was the explanation given by Anton herself for the ulceration. After she had been hit, a 'partial Tumor' had formed but had later disappeared.[49] Gregory saw fit to write down that Anton had for many years suffered from dyspeptic and hysterical complaints, which had alternated with an 'odematous affection of the left arm'. For this she had been admitted into the ward that winter, and had later been dismissed as cured of that complaint. At the time the breast had been medicated, but 'without benefit'.[50]

At the hospital, Anton was, it seems, given all possible care and treatment. Gregory carefully noted whether there was blood discharging from the breast or not and whether she suffered any pain. Thus we know that Anton was in pain on 20, 21, and 22 February, when she had more pain and 'very bad sleep'. This was repeated the next day, and on 24 February Gregory noted there was no change. On the 25th and 27th there was 'much more pain', and on the 28th there was 'great hemorrhagy' at night. This probably quite dramatic event received no other comment from Gregory, but the pain continued in March. Anton was given medication against pain throughout, but the pain evidently remained quite serious throughout her stay at the hospital. Some time in mid-March Gregory decided there was nothing more they could do, and Betty Anton, aged twenty-two, was released on 16 March.[51] Gregory scribbled down a blunt comment:

No change of symptoms.
Goes out without relief.[52]

Christie McKenzie's case has similarities to Anton's case. When she was admitted, 'a constant obtuse Pain' was troubling her in the middle of her sternum, and she suffered from a severe cough. Gregory noted that this cough 'exites an acute Pain under the right Breast'. McKenzie reported to Gregory that the pains had come a year earlier 'in consequence of lifting a weight', and that she had suffered from cough for two years. She said she had not used any medicines, which to me seems atypical.[53] She continued much the same during her first days at the hospital, but towards the end of March her breast was suppressed further, as was her cough, and at times she was further troubled by thirst, anorexia and costiveness. Up till then her case might have been considered one of consumption, but on 30 March a severe erythema[54] appeared on her left breast and spread rapidly. In only two days it reached her back. On 2 April, Gregory noted, there was a 'pretty large gangrenosis on ye lower half of the left Mamma'.[55] Medicated, McKenzie slept at night rather well and without delirium, which apparently had earlier troubled her. From 7 April onwards her gangrenous sore on the breast spread, and she was probably in great pain, since Gregory prescribed her some opiates for the night. On the 10th the erythema was better but the gangrene separated with copious discharge.[56] Here Gregory's notes on McKenzie come to an abrupt end. There is space for him to continue recording her case,[57] but for some reason the case was never closed. This was not customary for Gregory. The omission of the end of McKenzie's case is quite exceptional, and for our purposes more than unfortunate; we are left without any knowledge of her fate, although hoping that she improved.

These two cases nevertheless reveal that pain was an important message to the physician: it gave him hints of the patient's state and helped to direct the medicating process. In McKenzie's case the medication helped her to sleep, and probably allowed her to gather some strength, but this did not prevent her condition from worsening. Sleep, however, gave hope: the possibility that when a patient gained strength by sleeping she would be able to improve.

In Barbara Hanawalt's words, '[n]othing can be more spatially confining than enforced silence in which the very escape of words puts the speaker in a marginal category'.[58] One may assume that early modern breast cancer patients, at least toward the end of their illness, were suffering something similar. As we have seen, even early phases of the disease could produce such pain that any rest, let alone sleep, was impossible. This was often reiterated, and Mrs Elliot from Wormley Bury, Hertfordshire is typical in this sense:

> [T]here were five large ulcers discharging an exceedingly offensive matter, excrescences were likewise forming and sloughing away continually. This disorder had been had nine months. The pains were acute, and the matter discharged was so corrosive, as to erode the adjacent parts. Neither ease nor rest could be obtained even by the use of opiates.[59]

The nature of cancer pain was total. The body withered, and the mind suffered perhaps even more. As John Ewart recorded his patient's Susan Alford's condition:

> Her appetite and strength were much impaired, her body had been progressively emaciating, and her spirits were sunk with long suffering, and the despair of finding relief. She complained of attacks of shivering, succeeded by heat and thirst, and afterwards by cold sweats, which particularly occurred in the night.[60]

Because of the pain, Alford had been forced, six years earlier, to give up her profession as cook. Her illness, as Ewart put it 'rendered her unable to follow her profession', as moving the arm on the side of the diseased breast gave her severe pain.[61] Losing her livelihood alone was devastating, and the horrible effects of the illness added to her sufferings. Ewart takes care to be exact and use his patient's own words, and he gives a direct quote from Susan Alford: her pains were *'as if burned by live coal+'.* At the bottom of the page he explains the symbol '+': '+ Her own expression'.[62] This meticulousness reflects his need to convey to his readers the patient's terrible experience and the desperate state she was in, so as to convince them that the subsequent cure occurred with a person who was severely ill. I am inclined to believe this indeed is a direct quote from Susan Alford, and consider this a rare glimpse into the expression of the pain felt by a woman with an ulcerated breast. A cook by profession, Alford knew very well what it felt like being burned by a coal. The metaphor conveyed her experience with precision. Ewart used other direct quotes from Mrs Alford, all of which had to do with life in the kitchens: the growth on her breast resembled *'an unripe mulberry'*;[63] the circumference of her fissure was 'a small tea-cup'; while the hardened base was 'a large tea-saucer'.[64] Susan Alford's case shows that patients tried to make their illness and sufferings understandable to others, and that the experience of suffering could in fact be conveyed. These suffering women expressed their illness in terms that were familiar and understandable in their culture. The most horrible pain could be expressed to others, if not always in so many words, or with expressions as precise as those of Susan Alford; perhaps in multiple screams. Even if the audience was unable to imagine exactly how the patient felt, they were probably able to imagine enough. In this sense, utter bodily pain was communicable, and we can allow for outsiders' empathy.[65]

To remain with Susan Alford, Ewart mentions that she screamed: 'The whole was attended with almost constant pricking pain, which she sometimes compared to a sensation of burning; and this frequently increased to such an extreme degree of agony as to make her scream out for hours together'.[66]

Fanny Burney's Scream

Fanny Burney screamed from pain during her mastectomy. She did not remain silent; her pain was expressed. Before her operation, Burney's surgeons asked her if she had screamed when her son Alexander was born. Scholars have been unable to explain conclusively why Burney was asked this in the first place,[67] but if we look at her text carefully, it provides an answer. It is a simple one, but it is adequate, and logical:

> M. Ribe had *charged* me to cry! to withhold or restrain myself might have seriously bad consequences, he said. M. Moreau, in ecchoing [*sic*] this injunction, enquired whether I had cried or screamed at the birth of Alexander - Alas, I told him, it had not been possible to do otherwise; Oh then, he answered, there is no fear![68]

The answer as to why Burney was asked if she cried is to be found in Roselyne Rey' brisk notion:

> The notion that a sensation should be expressed by cries and moans followed the same model as that governing unwholesome humours and tainted, retained blood; it involved the same logic that led to excising a wound, to encouraging suppuration and to giving vent to pain.[69]

Thus, not to cry when in terrible agony was dangerous. Crying vented the body, eased the pressures inside it. It was understood to be possible that pain could kill a patient, and crying could thus save a life.[70] Furthermore, for the surgeon pain was a diagnostic tool, but it also helped him to determine what was possible to do and what was not.[71] To cry out was healthy, and that is what Burney did when she was operated on.

Thus her pain and suffering was vented by her screams, but it also gave her pain an expression:

> Yet – when the dreadful steel was plunged into the breast – cutting through veins – arteries – flesh – nerves – I needed no injunctions not to restrain my cries. I began a scream that lasted unintermittingly during the whole time of the incision – & I almost marvel that it rings not in my Ears still! so excruciating was the agony.[72]

Regarding Fanny Burney's mastectomy, Kay Torney has observed a gradual word-lessness which enters into Burney's account when she describes her mastectomy:

> she finds more that is sayable in analysing and complaining about the world of her doctors' ethical problems and her observation of the gap between their feeling for her as a person and a patient, than about her pain. The worse the pain gets, the more the sufferer is forced into wordlessness or into making the sort of noise that only conveys the bald information that pain is being felt. A writer who wants to describe a painful experience will be forced to 'code' it, finding ways of putting the wordless into language, and may rely on social and medical 'extras' as a way into wordlessness.[73]

To some extent I can agree with this interpretation. Burney's account does not give away a woman who would shut into total silence, but she herself makes this interpretation available, through her use of such words as 'a terror that surpasses all description' or 'speechless torture'.[74] Even for the husband, the operation and the hours following it were too horrible to describe: 'No language could convey what I felt in the deadly course of these seven hours'.[75] These screams were a release from pain but also a form of communication: to reach the people in the room, perhaps to signal even to oneself that one was alive.

Elaine Scarry has noted that '[p]hysical pain does not simply resist language but actively destroys it, bringing about an immediate reversion to a state anterior to language, to the sounds and cries a human being makes before language is learned'.[76] Scarry considers immense physical pain to be beyond everyday language; interestingly, however, she notes that sufferers reverts to the 'sounds and cries' we make before we learn to express ourselves in words. Fanny Burney would have agreed. She never pretended pain could be described fully in writing, even though she was a skilful author. In that sense there was a silence, even in the midst of her terrible scream. Pain indeed could be 'too severe to be contained within languages', as David Morris puts it.[77] Metaphors were needed. This context is of course the culture in which the patient lived, communicated and participated, and her pain is therefore only understandable through the metaphors she uses to describe her experience. Susan Alford's hot coals are a perfect example of these necessary metaphors.[78]

Jeremy Collier interestingly noted that utmost pain closed off one's senses, and that this was an act of God's mercy:

> God has so mercifully order'd the case, that the Extremity of Torment should quickly break the Sences, and extinguish the Punishment. Nay sometimes in the height of a Fever, when the Veins are all on fire; when the occasional Causes of Pain are most active and formidable; the Soul is as it were taken aside, and the Feeling laid asleep for a little time: Just as if a Man should have a friendly pull out of a House when part of it was tumbling, and not suffer'd to go in till 'twas better repair'd. To lie thus under shelter till the Storm of the Disease is somewhat over is next to a Miracle of Mercy in the Make of us.[79]

This is something we might call a shock reaction, a merciful reaction, which momentarily blocks out one's senses. Accounts of pain being numbed, however, are virtually non-existent. As we have seen, the accounts generally describe extreme pain. Such was for a long time the condition of Frances Day, lacemaker, from Goldington, near Bedford.[80] In 1813, when she was about nineteen years old, she had to enter the Bedford Infirmary because of the trouble and extreme pain a lump in the centre of her right breast gave her. She was advised to have the breast removed surgically. She was tormented, and had been so for years. She told Young that she had first noticed her lump when she was fourteen. Young mentions that the girl had been naturally full-breasted. For three years the lump gave her no trouble, but when she was seventeen 'her constitution first altered'.[81] The breast swelled and became painful, impeding her work as lacemaker. The lump had grown from its original size of a marble to that of an egg, and it 'in particular disturbed her'. The lump got worse, and apparently grew even larger; she then observed some soft substance growing out of the top of the hard lump. Young observes that she noticed this change promptly, as she was 'frequently induced to examine the lump and breast, for the pain she suffered'.[82] At the age of seventeen this is hardly surprising. She was at an age when she was supposed to be at her best, and was undoubtedly suffering not only from the pain caused by the lump but also from fears aroused by the unusual changes in her body. I have no great doubt that she would not have feared the worst – a cancer.

But pain followed her. As we have seen, Day was now in constant pain. We do not know if she saw any physicians or apothecaries at this time, although she probably asked the advice of other women, perhaps her mother, and tried some of the recipes that as we have seen were readily available. What we do know is that if she did attempt a cure, it did not give her any release from either the growth or the pain. The lump enlarged, 'till at length, in the winter, 1813, she was advised to go into the Bedford Infirmary.'[83] It was probably an apothecary, a physician or a clergyman that urged her to go to the hospital; these are the professionals she might have turned to when the situation became unbearable.

In the winter of 1813 Frances went to the Infirmary. Being a young woman she was probably taken there by a relative, but despite the comfort of being with a familiar person the place might not have much eased her pain and fear. One wonders if she thought she might not walk out of there alive. Or perhaps she was in too much pain to think about much else. Perhaps the building made no impression on her because of the pain.

What happened inside the hospital is decipherable from the few words Young gives us: 'The disease was being considered cancerous, an operation was proposed, to which she could not make up her mind to submit, and at length came out'.[84] She was not given any good news. Here one cannot but try and sense the confusion and fear this information must have given her. She refused the operation, 'to which she could not make up her mind to submit'.[85] We can, again, only guess: did she refuse the operation because she did not want to be mutilated? After all, she was so very young; perhaps she hoped to be able to marry one day, and have children. Did she think of the operation as a last resort, and that it was not time for it yet? Was she simply too frightened of the horrible operation, unable to face the unbearable pain it would cause? Was she afraid the operation would kill her? Any or all of these may contributed to her decision.

Since Young says that *at length* she came out of the hospital, she probably stayed there for some kind of treatment for a fairly prolonged period of time. It might have been a few weeks, as in the case of Betty Anton in the Edinburgh Infirmary. She too left the hospital bed in an open-ended situation; as we recall, her doctor noted in his diary: 'Goes out without relief'.[86] Similarly, in the winter of 1813 Day, lacemaker, had to return home to Goldington from the Bedford Infirmary, probably not having received much relief from her pains. She might have been given some painkilling medications, but she left the hospital with an illness she now knew was cancer.

According to Samuel Young, the specialists at the Bedford infirmary told her that her disease was cancerous.[87] They probably told her that the only way to cure her was to operate; as she refused, there was nothing she could do but leave. But she did search for help elsewhere. She certainly did not want to die young. She attended a quack, an 'empyrick', for six months, by which time her right arm was affected as well. By now her lacemaking was probably coming to a complete halt. In any case, she would have worked at home, just as so many other Bedfordshire women did, but the pain and the treatments would have made it very difficult for her to use her right hand.

Some time during the summer or autumn of 1813 she received an accidental blow to her breast, which further increased her sufferings. Young observes that during the time she was treated by the 'empyrick', she 'suffered a great deal of pain, which made her very ill indeed'.[88] This was a vicious circle: the medication made her condition worse by making her feel ill, probably nauseous and unwell.

When Frances Day first saw Samuel Young, he considered her case 'deplorable'. Grown to double its natural size, the whole breast was now under the strain of the illness: 'the fungus had rapidly increased, forcing the protruded integument almost to bursting. Drops, apparently of pure blood, fell from the nipple'.[89] Certainly Young felt sorry for this young woman. Her sufferings were apparent, even though she did not talk about them much; they were so plain that Young felt a need to convey them in his text: 'Naturally of a placid temper, she made no violent complaint; but her leaden complexion, and fixed abstracted countenance, were indicative of what she suffered'.[90] Day was withdrawn, perhaps distant, perhaps matter-of-fact, not there.

Yet Day continued her search for a cure or at least for relief. She came to Samuel Young for help. He gave her purgatives, mercurial alternatives[91] and leeches, which were attached to the side of the diseased breast, near the axilla. Her treatment continued until the spring, and she was alive when Samuel Young sent his manuscript to the publisher. He seems to have been certain that her story would have a happy ending. The breast would be removed: 'this case, placed under more favourable circumstances, would have ended before this, in an entire removal of the diseased parts; which there is not the smallest doubt will be finally accomplished'.[92]

Young thus seems to have agreed with the physicians and the surgeon of the Bedford Infirmary. They had been unable to persuade Day to have her breast removed; but perhaps, Young thought, she was now wiser. Perhaps she had already given hints that she would now agree to be operated on. She would be cured, he was sure. We are told no more of her fate. It is comforting that I cannot find a female death under Day's name in the records for the years following 1815.[93] Present-day knowledge about cancer suggests that her condition most likely was not cancerous, and she probably survived. Even if she agreed to surgery, she may have lived quite a happy life after recovering from the operation.

Where Day's experience remains much a mystery to us, her namesake D'Arblay, better known as Fanny Burney, gave a detailed account of her mastectomy. In our efforts to understand how such an operation was experienced, Burney's account is of unique and crucial importance.

Since Fanny Burney's breast was considered fully infected with cancer, her mastectomy was quite radical. According to her, her operation – including treatment and dressing – lasted a full twenty minutes. It was pure torture. She writes from Paris to her sister and others back home in England:

> My dearest Esther, – & all my dears to whom she communicates this doleful ditty, will rejoice to hear that this resolution once taken, was firmly adhered to, in defiance of a terror that surpasses all description, & the most torturing pain. Yet – when the dreadful steel was plunged into the breast – cutting through veins – arteries – flesh – nerves – I needed no injunctions not to restrain my cries. I began a scream that lasted unintermittingly during the whole time of the incision – & I almost marvel that it rings not in my Ears still! so excruciating was the agony. When the wound was made, & the instrument was withdrawn, the pain seemed undiminished, for the air that suddenly rushed into those delicate parts felt like a mass of minute but sharp & forked poniards, that were tearing the edges of the wound – but when again I felt the instrument – describing a curve – cutting against the grain, if I may so say, while the flesh resisted in a manner so forcible as to oppose & tire the hand of the operator, who was forced to change from the right to the left – then, indeed, I thought I must have expired. I attempted no more to open my Eyes, – they felt as if hermetically [sic] shut, & so firmly closed, that the Eyelids seemed indented into the Cheeks. The instrument this second time withdrawn, I concluded the operation over – Oh no! presently the terrible cutting was renewed – & worse than ever, to separate the bottom, the foundation of this dreadful gland from the parts to which it adhered – Again all description would be baffled – yet again all was not over, – Dr. Larry rested but his own hand, & – Oh Heaven! – I then felt the Knife <rack>ling against the breast bone – scraping it! – This performed, while I yet remained in utterly speechless torture, I heard the Voice of Mr. Larry, – (all others guarded a dead silence) in a tone nearly tragic, desire every one present to pronounce if any thing more remained to be done; The general voice was Yes, – but the finger of Mr. Dubois – which I literally *felt* elevated over the wound, though I saw nothing, & though he touched nothing, so indescribably sensitive was the spot – pointed to some further requisition – & again began the scraping! – and, after this, Dr. Moreau thought he descerned a peccant attom, – and still, & still, M. Dubois demanded attom after attom.[94]

What the reader first and foremost notices in this description is Fanny Burney's pain. For us it is inconceivable that one could survive a mastectomy without anaesthesia, but Burney forces us to believe that she did so. She felt pain but she also felt scraping; it seems that it was not only the pain but the operation itself that she felt. She was not numb.

Autobiographies and first-person novels were especially important reading matter in the eighteenth century, but had become so already in the previous century, when spiritual autobiographies and diaries in particular were very popular.[95] We must read Fanny Burney's autobiographical account of her mastectomy as a narrative of pain, both mental and physical.[96] It is some sort of irony that her letter concentrates on the immense pain caused her by the twenty-minute operation, that her experience is epitomized in those minutes; in fact, her pain actually lasted for months. The post-operative pain resulting from the operation rendered her life extremely difficult, and this included writing. Burney wrote her account months after her ordeal, and even then special arrangements had to be made for her to be able to use her hand in writing.

To us these sufferers were quite heroic in their pursuit of survival, but it is not only we who consider their strength great; the contemporaries of these patients agreed with us. Next, I take a look at the early modern spectator, friend and relative, and his or her views of the sufferers. What dominates the discussion is the great heroism of women who suffered from the ravages of cancer in their breasts.

Heroes of the Greatest Kind?

It is only natural that there were many ways to react to suffering, to pain and to the horrors of a mastectomy. One way to look at the sufferer was with admiration and respect. Since most of us have an understanding of what severe pain is like, it is probably only natural and human that we tend to consider those who suffer the greatest pains as actually heroic.[97] Porter and Porter suggest that early modern people too respected those who suffered pain: it was especially 'admirable to bear pain with fortitude'.[98] Since cancer was understood to be a cause of terrible pain, cancer patients were generally treated with awe and admiration: their sufferings made them heroic. For women this was an occasion to show fortitude, a trait which more often was attributed to the male sex.

David Morris has noted on the nature of pain that 'Pain on occasion becomes the site of encounters we can do nothing except witness in respect'. While many modern authors have stressed the ways in which sufferers are made admirable, we can also pay more attention to what Morris says: the reaction of a witness to suffering can be nothing but respect – and the sufferers, he comments, often 'move along us with a kind of holiness'.[99] Without romanticizing pain or the sufferer, I am tempted to treat the early modern observer from a somewhat similar position: he or she had little choice but to admire those who had to undergo pains that were universally accepted as being of the utmost horror. We should not necessarily see artifice in the process of heroification. Let us see why.

The pains of a woman with cancer were so formidable that they worked well in situations where metaphors for the most extreme form of suffering were needed. Richard Steele, describing the religious duties of ageing persons, listed repentance as the 'First Work of Old-age'; repentance, he wrote, was a 'bitter Pill' but if it was not taken, the pains of eternity would not be as the labouring woman's. God supported her, and to carry her further there was also the remembrance of the wonderful outcome of that particular pain: the child. If the 'bitter Pill' of repentance were not taken, the pains would be worse than the 'gnawing pains' suffered by a woman with cancer: they would be 'infinitely sharper, and infinitely longer'.[100] It is interesting that the most horrific pains described here are represented as specifically feminine pains: those of childbirth and of female cancer. It was of course the woman's lot to suffer; femininity brought specific pains, which were accepted as being extreme.[101]

It is possible that the heroic nature of the sufferers sprang from the cultural idea that human beings were supposed to suffer from the coils of this world. As Roy Porter put it, 'suffering was *everyone's* lot sooner or later, low- or high-born'.[102] It was heroic to suffer in a noble manner, and to meet the human lot with as much dignity as possible. It is perhaps pessimistic to suggest, following Elaine Crane, that women were expected to suffer more than men, and in silence, because they had to show submission to God's will,[103] but this rings true to a certain extent. These expectations did not mean, however, that women did not often resist them. A great determination to fool death and diminish suffering was for many an important target. At times, and for some patients, resignation was the best choice: to give up resistance, and submit to death. Such resignation is what we can read from the evidence given by Henry Slingsby, whose wife probably died of breast cancer:

> she was exceeding timerous, & fearefull; which made her apprehend many dangers to her self; she would say she was not affraid to dye, but of ye pains of Death; & to her physitian she would say, she desir'd nothing to prolong her life, so she could have any thing to ease her pains; so it happn'd to her as she fear'd, for certainly she dy'd a very painful death, having ye use of her speech & senses & memory to ye very moment she dy'd; now what loss is to be compar'd to my loss?[104]

Although her husband considered her a fearful woman, Mrs Slingsby feared physical pain more than dying, and that fate seems to have been exactly what happened to her: a painful and probably prolonged death. Like many patients who died of breast cancer, she too remained conscious probably until very near death. In early modern theory it was natural to assume one could bring on an illness by fearing it.[105] Henry Slingsby seems to have been quite understanding of her wish to die instead of having to suffer prolonged, horrible pains, and when she finally is released from the pain, he considers her fortunate – he is the one suffering the greatest loss, as he now has to live without his wife. Even such a decision could be considered courageous, and interpreted – in religious terms – as making acceptable haste towards the pleasures of heaven.

Courage

Courage and strength were common themes in various accounts of breast cancer, especially in the eighteenth century. The anonymous author of *Ode to Melancholy* (1782), written 'to the memory of a lady who died of a cancer in the breast', emphasized the lady's strength during moments of pain. She was a heroine of the greatest sort, and she dared to live in this world:

> Mother of Musings, hear me tell
> How valued, and how wept she fell;
> How great, how good, and how serene
> She liv'd superior to the sense of pain.
>
> By Reason's and Religion's aid,
> In keenest tortures undismay'd,
> She own'd unerring Wisdom's hand,
> And bow'd obedient to this dread Command.
>
> Oppression knew not to controul
> Her native dignity of foul;
> Unmov'd her conscious virtue bore
> The fiercest shocks of Fortune's tyrant power.
>
> With more than female tenderness,
> She triumph'd ev'n amid distress;
> With more than manly fortitude,
> Look'd up to Heaven, and 'saw that all was good'.
>
> 'Midst every hope and comfort lost,
> A CHRISTIAN'S name was all her boast:
> This could all other wants supply,
> By this she dar'd to live, nor fear'd to die.[106]

This woman and her fortitude seemed to conquer death, with her Christian faith to exceed most human beings and human qualities. She was above pain and torture, overcame her feminine weaknesses, and with more 'manly fortitude' reached heaven with her acceptance of her faith and willed afterlife. She was fearless, a true heroine, untainted by her decaying breast. Clearly, exceptional circumstances gave an exceptional, courageous woman a chance to cross the dividing line between the sexes. Moreover, in distress she could have more than 'manly fortitude' – she could be like a man, indeed more than a man. Situations like this offered women a chance to transcend boundaries, to be an ideal human being. Early modern gender was fluid.

Manly fortitude was especially needed when one decided to have a surgical operation, and it is not surprising that heroism presents itself in accounts of mastectomies. It must have been a difficult choice for patients to make; as Henry Fearon puts it, 'it requires a greater degree of resolution than most of them can readily summon up, to submit to it'.[107] Those who did were admired for their fearlessness.

In Stratford-upon-Avon in 1666, Mrs Townshend had a mastectomy. We know of it because the Reverend John Ward reported it in his diary.[108] Mrs Townshend was Ward's parishioner, and it was by no means unusual for a cleric to have been present and assisting at such operations; many clergymen practised medicine to some extent in their parishes. When Mrs Townshend, unaided by the operation, later died of breast cancer, Ward was present at her dissection as well. He makes a point of Mrs Townshend's tenacity. He reports that the doctors and surgeons considered her capable of enduring the knife; in her case, the operation was considered a good choice. Ward further notes that one of the surgeons (he neglects to mention his name, but it was either 'Clerk of Bridgnorth' or 'Leach of Sturbridg'),[109] after the mastectomy, had told Mrs Townshend 'that shee had endured soe much, that hee would have lost his life ere hee would have sufferd the like'.[110] The surgeon went on to say that 'hee had read that women would endure more than men, but did not beleeve itt till now'.[111] The surgeon's surprise was understandable, as women were usually seen as the weaker vessel. On the other hand, there was an understanding that women were oppressed with great woes, especially relating to the burdens of childbirth, and that they were tenacious. Mrs Townshend's conduct suggested to the surgeon that what he had heard really was true: what he saw proved to him that he, as a man, could not have come out of the experience alive.

Jeremy Collier analysed the reasons why women might endure more than men: 'Women used to Sickness will bear the Fatigues of it better than Men of a healthy Constitution. How comes this to pass? Are the Organs worn up, and stupified? Or is the Mind grown callous by being accustomed to Blows, and battering?'[112] Collier suggests that women were more used to being ill than men, and perhaps even used to being ill-treated. Women, of course, were understood to have been cursed because of Eve's sin to suffer pain, especially in childbirth; thus suffering was in a way their lot. Much of this suffering occurred hidden away from men's eyes – the childbed for example was women's own space, to which men had no access;[113] but a disease such as breast cancer could not go unnoticed or behind closed doors. Visible suffering could thus surprise men greatly, and make women great heroes in men's eyes.

William Cowper depicts in his manuscript casebook the case of a Mrs Woaden, who was operated on 13 April 1698. He seems to have appreciated her courage greatly; he considered it worth mentioning that 'She came to the Operation with as much Courage I ever saw'.[114] Mentioning the patient's courage was by no means strictly germane in a brief depiction of a surgical operation, thus giving his words even greater weight.

Cowper was assisted by two surgeons; while he himself first put his hand on the tumour, Mr Guddier (Goodyear?) thrust his hamulus (a needle-like hook) into the breast and used it to pull the tumour towards himself. Cowper then 'separated ye morbid p[ar]t' with six strokes.[115] This was normal procedure in amputations, and undoubtedly required courage; of which in Cowper's assessment, as we have seen, Mrs Woaden had more than most.

Mrs Woaden may have shown similar courage to Mary Astell who, if we are to trust George Ballard's account of her operation, chose to remain completely quiet about her disease and her operation and who remained quiet during her operation. The female author emerges as the great, courageous heroine of a novel:

> She seemed so regardless of the sufferings or pain she was to undergo, that she refused to have her hands held, and did not discover the least timidity, or impatience, but went thro' the operation without the least struggling or resistance; or even so much as giving a groan or a sigh: and shewed the like patience and resignation throughout the whole cure, which that gentleman, to his lasting credit and honour, soon performed.[116]

In this account, what seems to be important is her resignation to go through with the operation, without many people to assist or anyone else to observe – and to be stoic throughout the operation itself. Ballard points out that she did not want to have her hands held; but it seems inconceivable that any surgeon would have began a surgical operation without ensuring the patient could not do further harm to herself.[117]

Mr Johnson also operated on Lady Betty Hastings's breast. Her biography, by Thomas Barnard, was published in 1742. Lady Betty was a very well-known character in her time, and in the context of biographical writing it is hardly surprising that she was depicted as the epitome of courage and heroism. According to Barnard, she met the illness without any complaints, and continued her normal life up to the day of her operation. Her stoicism was admirable, considering that she was a close friend of Mary Astell, who only a few years earlier had succumbed to breast cancer.[118] When the moment of the operation came, she sat 'loose and indifferent for Life or Death'.[119] Her fortitude was astonishing to Ballard: 'her Hands were held by Men of Strength; – her Hands might have been held by Spider's Thread; no Reluctancy did She show, no Struggle, or Contention or even any Complaint did She make'.[120] This might bring to mind the cultural 'must' of female subjection, but we can also read this in another way. She was strong enough to subject herself to this torture. After the operation, Lady Betty surprised everyone by recovering more quickly than expected. She returned to her normal life for a while, to help others and to serve God.[121] When her death was imminent she put her energy to helping others; she wrote a great number of letters to help and give counsel; and – perhaps the greatest sacrifice of all – she had to stay alive for more than a year after the date of her will. In that she succeeded.[122] Lady Betty Hastings met her illness and her fate, of death from cancer;[123] it was her relationship with God and religion which Barnard – and probably Lady Betty herself as well – interpreted as the source of her fortitude and courage.[124]

Alexander Pope wrote an epitaph for a Mrs Corbet with the title 'On a lady, who died of cancer in her breast':

Here rests a woman, good without pretence,
Blest with plain reason, and with sober sense:
No conquest she, but o'er herself desir'd;
No arts essay'd, but not to be admir'd.
Passion and pride were to her soul unknown,
Convinc'd that Virtue only is our own.
So unaffected, so compos'd a mind,
So firm, yet soft, so strong, yet so refin'd,
Heaven, as its purest gold, by tortures try'd,
The saint sustained, but the woman dy'd.[125]

To Pope, the lady's suffering was saintly indeed, the spirit endured, but the tortured body, the woman, had to give in. Pope speaks directly of the tortures she had to go through. Samuel Johnson admired this epitaph, noting that he had 'always considered this as the most valuable of all Pope's epitaphs'.[126] It was reprinted in various anthologies, and was undoubtedly considered an exemplary work; a death from breast cancer called for such lines, expressing admiration of female heroism.

I have not intended here to argue that *all* women were in fact great heroines and silent sufferers. What I am arguing is that the cultural image of these sufferers formed and articulated them as such; but, it must be noted, it also provided a space for women who acted in a more unruly manner. As we have seen, many women were stubborn patients, and knew what they wanted no matter what their surgeons and physicians thought. Their unruliness could take many forms. Jane T's operation went well, and she was put to bed after having had her wound dressed. Later, however, her surgeon, James Nooth, found her using her arm, which he had clearly advised against – and which in his eyes was dangerous:

on calling to see her in the evening, I found her actually employing it in repairing some part of her dress. I made her sensible of her unwarrantable deviation from my advice, but I had no reason afterwards to charge her with imprudence.[127]

He mentions that she was repairing her dress. Was she actually sewing? If so, one would like to think that in her case at least the painkillers were effective. This case brings to mind the feminine ideal of keeping occupied: it was not appropriate to be idle, and some needlework or mending would be quite a suitable occupation for a woman of Jane T.'s age and class. Perhaps she was repairing her dress so as to accommodate her dressed breast more comfortably, because she was concerned about causing irritation to her chest.

A different kind of unruliness is found in the case of a middle-aged woman who had just weaned her child when Norford saw her for her worrisome, knotted, itchy breast with a tumour. He introduces her as 'the Mother of several Children, subject to nervous Complaints, and a little addicted to the Drinking of spirituous Liquors'. When, he continues, 'I prescribed her a cooling Diet, but she did not observe my Directions so well as she should have done; only in the Room of Brandy, which sometimes she mixed with a little Water, and drank at her Meals, she now condescended to drink White-Wine and Water'.[128] To a brandy drinker, switching from brandy to white wine must have been quite a concession.

Naturally, there is no way to arrive at absolute figures as to the number of women or the ways in which they reacted to their illness or to the treatment. To consider them human, fallible and suffering beings is only merciful. While the cultural idealization of a suffering woman seems to have been customary, it was probably not considered much out of the ordinary if a woman did not emerge victorious from her diagnosis. Alice Aris, who at the time she entered Dr Burrows's course of treatment was in the service of the family of the Duchess of Bridgewater, was unlike the women depicted earlier. She seems not to have taken the news of her terminal illness well. She became depressed. Let us allow John Burrows, M.D., to report the way in which he saw her:

> This patient, whose disorder proved to be of the most inveterate nature, was recommended to me in 1765, by some persons in the family of her grace the late Duchess of Bridgewater. She had already had the advice of several hospital surgeons, from whom receiving very little encouragement to hope for a cure, she became languid and extremely dejected.[129]

Burrows's treatment, however, worked for her, and she grew better: 'After these very promising symptoms, the patient grew daily more easy, recovered her rest in some degree, and her strength in a very short time, so far as to be able to attend daily at my house in order to be dressed'.[130] That she was 'languid and extremely dejected' speaks for her battered bodily and mental state: she became, in our terms, depressed, and had probably resigned herself to suffer horribly and die. Not everyone was a battling hero – and yet, even a woman with a languid and dejected mind could come through the disease.

Religion

Religion is an aspect we should not ignore in terms of female heroism in early modern self-understanding and overall interpretations of the sufferings of others. All in all, the role of religion in women's lives, while it was ever present, is discussed in women's diaries and letters in very subtle tones. Religion was often a given, which did not need to be explained in explicit terms; if, however, we look at different genres, and especially at funeral sermons and memoirs, it becomes clear that religion was an ubiquitous means for patients to understand the horrific turn their lives had taken. In memoirs religious interpretations of illness and suffering were frequently offered; religion was the means whereby such terrible events as a life-threatening illness were met, especially if one survived them. And after the patient's death, his or her religious nature was important to depict; these tales then become in a way travel narratives – journals of the process towards the great end, Heaven.

It was natural for others to write about a deceased person's religious piety and great suffering. This was an important cultural norm. Thomas Barnard praised the qualities of Lady Betty Hastings. In the same vein people made sense of the sufferings and death of one Mrs Elizabeth Moore in the mid-seventeenth century. Her illness left a trace which has reached us because her funeral sermon was printed. This sermon, and the memoirs already mentioned, may well overemphasize the piety and religiosity of Elizabeth Moore and other women, but they nonetheless offer us a valuable glimpse into the religious interpretation of this devastating illness.

The published version of the funeral sermon composed by Edmund Calamy reveals very little of Mrs Elizabeth Moore. It describes her as a poor woman, who throughout her life was 'loaded with many and great troubles'.[131] We know from the date of the book that she probably died some time around 1658. The writer mentions that she indeed died from a cancer in the breast,[132] and that 'her sickness was very long, and very painful':[133] her torments had lasted for more than a year, apparently three years, of which the last two were filled with pain.[134]

Unsurprisingly, Calamy's funeral sermon on Moore stressed that afflictions such as cancers were trials sent by God to test people. This meant that the person to be tested may have been one of His chosen. Moore wanted to show that those who suffered the most were by no means to be understood as having been the greatest sinners:

> when I see a godly woman afflicted, then I say, this is not so much for her sin, as for her trial; this is not to hurt her, but to teach her to know God, and to know her selfe, to break her heart for sin, and from sin, to make the world bitter, and Christ sweet. God hath put her into the fire of affliction, to refine her, and make her a vessel fit for his use. God is striking her with the hammer of affliction, that shee may bee squared, and made ready to bee laid in the heavenly Ierusalem.[135]

The sufferer was expected to take joy in God's trials. Mrs Moore is said to have found comfort in the thought that it was God who brought her her affliction: 'God picked her out to bee a pattern of afflictions'.[136] Calamy mentions that before her illness Mrs Moore had had great fears as to her salvation: she had always been God-fearing, but now her illness removed her timidity, 'all her doubts vanished'. According to Calamy she felt that she was especially chosen by God, which meant that there was hope of salvation for her.[137] To further emphasize her piety, Calamy mentioned that Elizabeth Moore wondered whether her particular heaven was in this life, since many people took 'compassion of her sad and afflicted condition', and contributed 'liberally towards her relief'. She was 'wonderfully comforted' by this.[138]

More than eighty years later, Lady Betty Hastings's biographer offered very similar interpretations. Barnard notes that 'the mighty torrent [of cancer was] ...

to solace her Spirit, and to strengthen her Assurance, that she had every Mark, and Token, of her Favour and Acceptance with God'.[139] She was heroic, believing herself to be God's instrument, especially in her patience, which grew when 'God increased her pains'.[140] Similarly too, Barnard notes of Lady Betty's heroism that it came from 'the true Spirit of his Religion'.[141]

Even though they lived in different centuries, the Christian role of the sufferer seems to have remained constant. Lady Betty Hastings wrote letters of great comfort to others, Moore's heroism was presented toward neighbours and friends in the form of oral advice. When people visited her, she gave counsel to them, and the author noted that

> I have heard her often, and often perswading her friends to prize health, and to improve it for the good of their souls, to lay up against an evill day, and to stock themselves with grace before sickness come. Shee would frequently say, O the benefit of health! O prize health! praise God for health, and improve health for your eternal good.[142]

Religion was a form of medicine for Mrs Moore and Lady Betty Hastings. Not was Moore in inward peace during her illness, she enjoyed God's consolations.[143] Lady Betty's afflictions were lightened by her great hope of Immortality.[144] Moore's special 'delight' was the Law of God: 'this kept her from perishing in her affliction. Shee was continually fetching cordials out of the Word, to comfort her under her great pains, and to preserve her from fainting'.[145] Faintings were a common danger for those who were under the great pains of cancer: by focusing on God's word, she was able to ease her pains and remain conscious. The author indeed speaks of cordials (wine and opium). In fact he mentions that it was Mrs Moore herself who had used this metaphor: 'shee said, that the Word of God was the best cordial in the world'.[146] Religion was literally Mrs Moore's opium.

As cancer in the breast was such a formidable enemy, it made a good religious *exemplum*. Calamy's sermon did not dwell on her death but stressed her influence on those around her during her life, both in illness and in health. This is exactly what Barnard did in his interpretation of Lady Betty's life: her imminent death is nothing compared to the glories of her actions, ensuring that her property would be distributed in a good way, and her great wish to help others, which led her to belittle herself and her sufferings.[147] In Moore's case, God gave the patient the long illness as a test: she sustained her faith through all the sufferings she was put to, not only by the illness itself but by all the treatments she received. She met these all with great patience: 'Shee would say, It was no matter; sanctified afflictions were better then unsanctified prosperity.'[148]

Two years of suffering of medicines and cautery, especially in the form of burning irons, added to Moore's sufferings an element which elevated her above ordinary women. Lady Betty Hastings, as a member of the elite, was of course in a different class, but she demonstrated her piety in similar terms. Both these women showed piety, as was customary and approved, even before their illness, but their cancer made them special. The author likens Moore's sufferings and death to martyrdom, so patient, meek and constant as she was – which of course was quite appropriate for a woman of no great position.[149] Lady Betty Hastings was portrayed as a formidable woman, strong enough to fool the lawmakers; but one who 'under this her sharp Chastisement' strove after all to serve others, as shown in her determination to endure the necessary days in order for her will to be valid.[150] Serving others was the way in which these women turned their horrendously difficult deaths to religious and pious victories. The pervasively Christian culture that surrounded them, in particular the Catholic tradition, had suggested to them models for managing pain, for welcoming suffering. The *Imitatio Christi* taught them to embrace illness and ordeals, to rejoice in them as a road to God.[151]

Empathy and Pity

Beyond great admiration and even heroification, onlookers also had other feelings towards those forced to suffer from cancer in the breast. Breast cancer was a disease which caused apprehension and great empathy even among professionals in the medical trade. This is reflected in contemporary medical ethics, in the way in which a good physician or surgeon met the patient and her sufferings.[152] But it was a given that people felt greatly for those close to them.

We know about the reaction of Dr Larrey, Fanny Burney's surgeon, to the prospect of her future mastectomy. Before the operation he was almost unbelievably reluctant to operate on her; afterwards he was in a deep state of grief – in Burney's words, 'pale nearly as myself, his face streaked with blood, & its expression depicting grief, apprehension, & almost horrour'.[153] Burney's account is embedded in early nineteenth century Romanticism and its 'sensibility', and we cannot perhaps extrapolate anything from it as to earlier reactions to mastectomies; but I tend to think that most surgeons felt for their patients, and some of them actually had to struggle to remain sufficiently detached to be able to perform the operation.

In Burney's case, it is fascinating to observe how much space she actually gives to the narrative of *her own* empathy and pity towards those who were close to her, especially her husband but also her son and her surgeon. She writes that she felt deeply for them, and wanted to keep her husband and her son as ignorant as possible of her true situation, the date of the operation and other excruciating facts.[154] We should keep in mind that even if a woman survived the operation and the spirit lived on, life after the operation was hardly easy. Fanny Burney gives us a first-hand account of this. Months after the operation she was still in deep pain: after the partial removal of her breast muscle writing was nearly impossible; even moving her hand was extremely difficult, and coughing and speech torturous: 'the oppression upon my breast makes all talking so fatiguing, so painful in its effect'. Even several years later, she felt she had not yet completely recovered.[155]

It seems to have been considered natural for the surgeon to feel for his patient during the operation. In order not to endanger the patient's life and the success of the operation, however, it was important to harden oneself against any plea from the patient. Any delay in an operation was dangerous. It was the surgeon's duty to remain calm and detached, ignoring the patient's pitiful cries:

> Many females can stand the operation with the greatest courage and without hardly moaning at all. Others, however, make such a clamour that they may dishearten even the most undaunted surgeon and hinder the operation. To perform the operation, the surgeon should therefore be steadfast and not allow himself to become disconcerted by the cries of the patient.[156]

A good surgeon was quick, thus preventing the prolongation of the patient's pain. This did not mean that any cruelty on the surgeon's part was accepted.[157] Especially notable in his empathy toward the patient was Pierre Dionis: he suggested that only one thrust of the needle was needed in inserting threads into the operated breast, he spoke of the need for speed in cutting, and he was sensible of the anguish of the patients over the general prognosis of cancer. He even suggests that surgeons should not introduce cautery irons into the room in which the operation was carried out, since 'these hot Irons make the Patient tremble' – and they were not actually of any use. Bleeding could be stopped by other means.[158] Dionis considered ulcerated cancer the worst of surgeon's challenges: not only did it trouble the patient, but 'nor is there any way which fatigues the Chirurgeon more, nor gives him more Trouble, because the Disease is almost always incurable'.[159]

In contrast, many case histories are devoid of expressions of pity or empathy toward the patient. This does not necessarily mean that the surgeon or the physician was completely cold towards the patient's sufferings. Rather, it may indicate that these sufferings were too self-evident to be worth mentioning. When Beckett for example writes about the forty-year-old woman, mentioned above, who died of breast cancer only three weeks after her operation, he has no words for her in describing the operation as such. On the other hand, in describing the situation preceding the operation, and especially her long sufferings with an ulcerated cancer, he reveals some empathy: the sore from which 'this poor Woman' suffered was 'very terrible'.[160]

William Rowley, as both a physician and a surgeon, seems throughout his *Seventy Four Select Cases* to be quite sympathetic towards his patients, who in many cases had suffered immense pains at the hands (according to Rowley) of incompetent quacks or colleagues who had been too eager to treat their tumours. One lady, for example, lingered, according to him, 'under the most distressing and accumulated miseries, shocking indeed to the spectators'.[161] Rowley had great empathy for his patients; one of his reasons for wanting to educate his colleagues so as not to try to heal breast cancer with caustic, acids, arsenic, bark or mastectomy seems to have been to spare the patient from such horrible pains. He viewed caustics, for example, as a 'barbarous treatment'.[162] Here his medical ethics, and his empathetic wish to save the patient from further harm, worked as an advertisement as well. It may have been a commercial ploy; but it nevertheless speaks of the cultural tenet that surgeons were supposed to be empathetic towards their patients and their sufferings. It is probably safe to argue that this empathy towards the patient was one reason why innovations occurred in the techniques of operating on the breast. Henry Fearon, for example, spoke strongly for saving as much skin or breast as possible and for suturing the lips of the wound in order to lessen the torture for the patient, since healing took much longer if the wound was left open.[163]

Cancer induced empathy even towards people whom one did not much like. In the late summer of 1766, Lady Mary Coke noted that Lady Waldegrave was ill, and that it was reported that the illness would be 'of a most terrible kind'. Undoubtedly this would have referred to a cancer, Lady Waldegrave had apparently had the complaint before, as Lady Mary Coke noted that it was 'thought the complaint has return'd in her breast'.[164] What Lady Mary is here reporting is of course – as she herself admits – merely a rumour circulating in polite society. Even as such, however, and even though the patient was clearly far from being her bosom friend, she felt great pity for Lady Waldegrave: 'tho' I think her a silly impertinent Woman, if the report is true, I pity her from the bottom of my heart'.[165]

Lady Mary returned to the topic of Lady Waldegrave's illness a little later. She had been given a report on her condition by Lady Tweedale, according to whom the illness had 'brought her [Lady Waldegrave] into a terrible condition, & that She was so greatly altered She had hardly the remains of beauty'.[166] These two sharp-tongued ladies then went on to wonder about the Duke of Gloucester's attachment to this woman, regardless of her illness or the loss of her beauty. Lady Tweedale had commented that 'in her condition, She was very Unfit for either Wife or Mistress'.[167] There remains not a trace of pity in these words, merely malice. Lady Mary Coke met Lady Waldegrave a few days later, in early October, and noted that she was not 'alter'd', but was 'thiner'.[168]

Lady Mary Coke, however, was once more full of empathy when she heard the bells toll for the funeral of Lady Cockburn. The latter had suffered from something extremely painful for months, and had eventually died. Lady Mary Coke reported thus:

> [A]s we passed Petershame Chapel the Bell was tolling for poor Lady Cockburn's funeral; I never heard of any person suffering such agonies as She did for seven months before it pleased God to release her; her torments were so great that She repeatedly begged of her Husband, in the most earnest manner, to put an end to her life, saying She was sure it cou'd be no sin.[169]

In such a case as this, it was surely considered a Christian thought to view death as a release, and I return to that point in concluding this chapter. By noting that Lady Cockburn had repeatedly asked her husband to terminate her miseries by killing her, Lady Mary corroborated the awful nature of the patient's pains. Lady Mary took no stance in the matter, but simply reported it; one wonders, however, if she considered such a request at least in part understandable.

'Much Desired, Welcome Death'

Dying from breast cancer was usually painful, more than painful. There were some cases, such as that of a certain lady of rank, where there was – at least according to William Rowley, who treated her – 'very little pain or no pain'.[170] More often, it seems, the case was completely different. From several accounts we learn that nothing seemed to help to relieve the pain, not even opiates. One such account tells the story of an unknown lady who died of breast cancer. She had tried various forms of treatment, most radically caustics, which might remove the cancerous growth; but they were felt to have aggravated her cancer, killing her far more quickly than the cancer would have done so had it been left alone. This lady's cancer spread to her other breast, and during the last weeks of her life she was in great agony. Even Rowley's somewhat laconic comments reveal something of the desperateness of her situation and the misery of dying:

> Sloughs succeeded sloughs, and occasioned a most offensive stench; the acrid discharge was considerable; the patient became hectical; opiates could not produce relief, and thus lingering under the most distressing and accumulated miseries, shocking indeed to the spectators, but inexpressibly so to the worthy lady who languished under them; she died about two months later.[171]

These agonies were so great, it seems, that at least during the latter half of the eighteenth century patients were regularly given opiates for relief. In 1698, Mrs Woaden, who as we recall was operated on by William Cowper, was given opiates after her operation for ten nights. This was clearly done to ease her sleep, and it seems to have helped in that respect.[172]

Often however, as in the unknown lady's case, even opiates were not enough to ease the pain.[173] This is what Jean Astruc is referring to when he mentions, in passing, the problems involved in the palliative care of breast cancers. Sometimes, he says, the cure is effective enough to prolong the patient's life, but at what a cost!

> It succeeds sometimes so far, as to prolong the patient's life; but they pay dearly for this delay, by suffering almost continual pains, which can only be moderated by the power of opium. I have often seen these pains brought to such an excess, that the patient has been compelled to consent to the extirpation, whatever repugnance she might have to it.[174]

In warning readers against succumbing to the enthrallment and wonderful promises of quacks, Henry Fearon offers the cautionary example of Mrs Chidley, from Pall Mall, who died after horrible suffering. She herself, according to Fearon, had wanted to publicize her story and her deception by a quack. He writes of her sufferings:

> For some time before her dissolution, the pain was at times so exquisite, that she would start out of bed and run about the house, up and down the stairs, like one frantic, though the ** weight of the tumor was so great that she had not strength even to sit up, except when seized with one of these fits. The smell at last was so offensive that it could be born only by those who had been accustomed to it from being constantly about Mrs. C.

The double asterisk in the quotation directs the reader to a footnote: 'The disease after her death being removed, weighed ten pounds and three quarters'.[175]

Since the pains of cancer meant suffering beyond the imagination, the death of the patient was often desired and welcomed, as noted by John Ball in *The Female Physician* (1770).[176] Above I have already briefly discussed the medical interpretation of a cancer death, and its horrible nature. Fearon calls the last stage of cancer 'that dreadful period which admits of no hope'.[177] It is important to remember that dying from a disease such as cancer was considered a natural death.[178] I next take a look at this death, and how it was met by both patients and their friends alike.

Early modern breast cancer, as said, was usually considered a death sentence. From a present-day perspective, the early modern breast-cancer patient had no chance of survival. In early modern terms, cancer was mostly seen as only rarely curable, although there was hope of postponing death for several years; but there were also those who thought a cure was possible.[179] As discussed earlier the view was often reiterated that if left alone, a cancer could be manageable for years. All in all, many were quite optimistic; but not many specialist surgeons who were consulted by cancer patients were this positive about the eventual possibility of prolonging life under such a threat. It was only to be hoped that God in his mercy would allow the sufferer to breathe her last.

The patient would be quite quickly consumed by cancer in the breast if the cancerous humours corroded the large vessels and there was much bleeding. Bleeding would make sure that 'the strength of the Patient is quickly spent, and the Spirits being exhausted and consumed, they soon dye'.[180] The significance of bleeding was recognized by the great authorities. Nisbet elaborated that in what we would call the terminal phase there were two specific killers. These were haemorrhage and convulsions, which would terminate 'a miserable and painful existence'.[181] Pearson too understood cancer to be lethal: '[t]he natural tendency of a Cancer, is to terminate in the certain destruction of those Patients that are unhappily afflicted with it'.[182]

Case histories often show that medical professionals left (allowed) their patients to die if their case was pronounced incurable and death imminent. This was not considered unfeeling or unethical. Rather, it reflects a very different view of the role for example of the physician: it was considered unethical to operate on a patient who had no chance of survival, as the operation would merely cause further pain. There were occasions when such operations were performed despite the hopeless state of the patient, in hope of easing the patient's sufferings.[183] As Andrew Wear notes, it was not until the end of the eighteenth century that the art of dying as a performance declined, after which it was possible for example to keep the patient in a sedated state by means of opiates. Earlier, the patient was expected to remain as clear-minded as possible, so as to be able to die according to the principles of a 'good death'. This is reflected in the roles that were assigned to physicians: death was not yet a medical but a religious event, an occasion between the dying person and God, not to be interfered with by medicine. If any professional was needed, it was a priest.[184]

To stop the disease from spreading, the treatment had to be quick. Mrs P., Dr William Rowley's patient died, according to him, because of her other doctors' and surgeons' incompetence in treating her disease correctly early on. When she was brought to him, it was already too late. Her surgeon had promised her a certain cure; but such promises were in Rowley's opinion vain, as he did not know the correct cure for the disease. Mrs P. had tumours in her breast and under her arm, which in our terms probably meant that her cancer was well advanced when she approached Dr Rowley. He could do nothing but mitigate her symptoms. She grew worse, had more and more difficulty in breathing, and finally died.[185] In the eighteenth century the process of the spreading of a cancer was familiar to physicians and surgeons. This left Rowley space to blame her other doctors, rather than admitting that her case had been quite incurable for a long time.

Pearson for example seems to have been well aware that a breast cancer could spread to the lungs. When he listed the conditions under which one should operate on a breast cancer, diseased lungs meant that there was no chance of an operation being beneficial: 'Or if from the presence of a cough, attended with difficult respiration, and expectoration of matter, and Hectick fever, there be reason to apprehend that the Lungs are in a diseased state, no particular is to be expected from the excision of the breast.'[186] There seems to have been a common understanding of the signs of a spreading cancer: the ill colour of the patient, and severe pains in the body, for example in the stomach.[187] Understanding the process of metastasis was naturally difficult without the concept of the cell. Ideas as to the process, however, were forming at least in the later part of the eighteenth century, promoted in part by clinical medicine and by specialists, who saw a large number of breast cancers and thus were able to recognize patterns in the behaviour of cancers. Jean Astruc, who considered maternal milk as the foremost and only cause of breast cancers, thought that it was a cancerous milk which moved towards the lymph nodes of the armpit and built obstructions there.[188] It would then obstruct the travel of lymph and blood to the arm; the arm would swell up, and its 'tumefied' state would hasten the patient's death.[189]

Le Dran wrote of the spreading of cancers, and accurately explained the process which sometimes took place:

> If, after a certain time, these swellings become painful, the *cancer* then commences, and in a short time probably the glands of the arm-pit are obstructed; in which case I have known fresh cancers to arise in different parts, even after the extirpation of that which appeared at first. In this case, the bones may break by being affected with the same cancerous humour.[190]

John Burrows believed that the problems and ulceration of the axillary lymph nodes was caused by the cancerous humour; he actually uses the term *metastasis*.[191]

Andrew Duncan among others considered it extremely important to halt the spreading of a cancer (or the cancer virus) by the knife. He spoke of 'absorption' as well as of the cancer virus spreading.[192] Richard Guy believed that absorption could occur even before the tumour turned malignant.[193] James Latta thought that cancer spread through absorption.[194]

John Hunter too had an idea of the process of metastasis: He believed it was matter absorbed from the tumour which caused the cancer to spread.[195] Let us take a closer look at one of Hunter's cases, which, to me seems pivotal in the history of understanding the nature of cancer.

Early modern doctors usually seem to have been aware that breast cancer often led to respiratory difficulties, including a severe cough.[196] For us respiratory problems immediately suggest that the cancer has metastasized to the lungs, while in early modern cases it was understood more as a consequence of the condition: but definitely as a sign that death was, if not imminent, inevitable.[197]

Mrs Ad—m was about forty years old when she observed a lump in her breast. A year later, in the autumn of 1792, the lump had grown considerably, and she came to see Hunter. He tried to stop its growth, at first with seeming success. However, he had grave doubts: 'I gave hints of my doubts about the Cure, and endeavoured to lead the mind to an operation.'[198] She apparently remained in his care until the following January, when she 'went into the Country', but her stay there was not long. In early February she returned to London, apparently because of the trouble her breast was giving her. The tumour had grown greatly, and – what was worse – there were signs of the cancer spreading.[199] For Hunter the tumour in the armpit, the cough, and the shortness of breath were empirical signs of the spread of the cancer. He duly observes that he has seen this 'often'. He explains the process, as said, as the matter from the Tumour being absorbed elsewhere. He blames the circulation of blood as the cause, but he could not be certain; he says that his ideas were 'only conjecture', simply because he had been unable to carry out autopsies of persons who had died of similar conditions.

But the case of Mrs Ad—m unfortunately changed that. Being in such ill condition, she 'now came to the resolution of having it removed'. But now Hunter himself was no longer willing to operate: he indeed feared the disease had spread, and that clearly the patient would not live long. In such a case it would have been quite unethical to operate. The patient and probably her relatives seem to have insisted, however, since Hunter notes that 'it was imagined that her cough and shortness of breathing was nervous'. The symptoms had appeared rapidly, and gave reason to believe that this might be the case.[200] Hunter gave way, and Mrs Ad—m had her breast and gland removed. Along with it came parts of her pectoral muscles, which were also 'found contaminated'. The operation went well and the wound healed, but the lung-based symptoms grew worse. She was not well, and with all her symptoms increasing, she died three weeks after the operation. John Hunter's chance to see inside the body improved: 'I wished to examine the body, which was allowed.'[201]

Hunter found Mrs Ad—m's lungs extremely diseased. There was

> disease *in* their substance... This disease was ... in form of Tumours; in larger quantity or masses in the mediastinum and anterior edge of the lungs where they adhered to the Mediastinum ... The substance of the lungs every where, was studded with them: some as small as peas, others as large as Walnuts, &c.[202]

The substance of these tumours was curious to him: they were soft and 'broke into pieces like a Jelly'.[203] To Hunter's mind, however, these tumours were too widespread to be completely explained by the absorption of cancerous matter.[204] The Hunterian collection apparently holds a sample of Mrs Ad—m's lung. Item P 190, reputed to be from her lungs, shows largish growths in the lungs. If the tumours indeed are histologically chondrosarcoma (a bone cancer), as is said, Mrs Ad—m probably suffered originally from bone cancer, which metastasized (not atypically) to the lungs; she may have had breast cancer as well. The rapidity of her death was probably due to these two simultaneous conditions. On the other hand, it is possible that P 190 is not after all Mrs Ad—m's lung.

Death from breast cancer was, as said, long and painful, and was in the end caused by bleeding or the failure of internal organs.[205] Mrs M., one of doctor Rowley's hopeless cases, died after prolonged suffering. Her disease had first appeared in the form of an indrawn nipple in 1767. She had consulted a surgeon, who had ordered an issue, and later some medications, including mercury pills. Rowley mentions that her illness did not worsen until 1771, when she was treated by a 'learned physician' with hemlock, a very popular medication at the time, and grew worse: the breast swelled and grew hard, and there were tumours under her arm. In 1772 her cancer was treated with caustics, which after a time removed the whole tumour. Two years went by, and small, pea-sized indurations appeared. From the latter part of 1774 to the spring of 1775 she was in great pain, and caustics were again applied to her growths. Rowley first came to examine her on 12 June 1775, at which time he told her relative that there was not much hope. His favourite medicines, incl. pilula rubra, seemed to help, however, and she grew quite well in only three months. As can be imagined, 'the lady went into the country happy beyond expression'; but she must have been disappointed beyond belief when the illness returned in less than a year in the form of ulcers. She suffered for two or three months, according to Rowley, before she died.[206] This would place the date of her death some time in December 1776, as she had improved within three months after Rowley began his treatments, i.e. in October 1775, and was then well for less than a year – perhaps until September 1776. She lived for two or three months, which would probably give December 1776 as the latest possible time of death. In other words, from the appearance of the first symptom – the indrawn nipple – she survived for ten years. Her cancer was clearly a slow type, apparently leading Rowley to wonder whether she might not have been spared altogether had she not been treated with caustics and the cancer had been left alone.

John Ball noted that the pains of ulcerated cancer were so enormous that death was a release, and long-awaited. The horror of the last stages of the illness is described by him in a manner which tells of experience:

> For when the skin is one broken, a dismal scene is opened, and nothing but a miserable death to be expected, the cancerous humour most greedily devouring the fleshy substance wherever it comes, and being of a caustic nature it corrodes and destroys the nerves and blood-vessels; from whence ensues a profuse loss of the vital fluid, and most commonly immoderate haemorrhages (fluxes of blood) conclude the doleful tragedy, bringing on their much desired and welcome death.[207]

Ball's book, from which this quotation is taken, was intended in particular for a female readership, and his frankness reveals a need to be informative, truthful and perhaps empathetic.

In the end, what remained was indeed only death. 'The cup of the sufferer', as Nisbet eloquently put it, was not filled with hope, 'the only solace of the wretched'. Hope was 'banished' from her cup. This 'formidable malady' made certain that 'every patient, therefore, under this disease, may be viewed as consigned to a slow, painful, and lingering death, without hope of alleviation'.[208]

EPILOGUE

Death from breast cancer is rarely serene and beautiful. As a historian, I feel and have felt extremely uncomfortable relating the horrendous sufferings of these patients; yet I would feel equally uncomfortable omitting them, leaving my reader with the image of a sweet and pleasant death. Cancer in the breast was a greatly feared disease, and with good reason. It tortured the patients, often for years, by its pricking and darting pains, by ulceration, and by the slow progress of the disease in general.

The treatments of today's cancers are often described as barbarous, and I have oftentimes been reminded by today's cancer patients not to underestimate the horrendous, painful and nauseating nature of cancer medicine of our own day. Understanding this makes a scholar humble, and further helps us to understand the past realities: whatever the time of history, illnesses such as cancer are nothing but terrible. And it does not make sense comparing the experiences of patients from different centuries.

Eighteenth-century treatments of cancer were built upon ancient tradition, new ones were developed with the interest, I believe, of all humankind in mind: it was too well understood that cancer could, in fact, be an enemy to anyone, regardless of his or her status in the world or his or her way in the world. The eighteenth century saw new techniques in surgery, and many, I believe, greatly benefited from the early radical mastectomies, closing the wound at the first intention, or the newly recovered carrot poultice. Cancer remains much a mystery today, and it was more so to the eighteenth-century men and women, but as today, even then many eagerly sought a cure, and a valid explanation for the illness.

The ravages of cancer moved compassion, and raised disgust. Cancer was repulsive. While ideal beauty was seen as perfect harmony, breast cancer worked against that by growing mass which was out of the ordinary and out of place. The breast with cancer often burst open, ulcerated, when the tumour grew, and it leaked ill smelling, nauseating, fluids. This with the pains the illness caused, raised great empathy in people who attended the patient, including the medical professionals.

The patients, even if in their last weeks of life, typically remained adamant that they wanted to do something about their illness. They were unwilling to give in, and many wanted to have surgical operations at very late stages of their illness. This reflects the early modern notion of the patient as the determining agent of his or her treatment: the patient still was the agent of her life. She decided her own treatment, and she eagerly shopped for the best cure.

While we cannot say how common cancer in the breast was in the eighteenth century, we can safely say that it was understood to be common. Everyone seemed to know someone with it, and patients shared recipes as well as information on the best and most resourceful and successful healers. Cancer devastated lives, killed too many at too early a stage. It was a devious illness, abhorred and detested as it disfigured, tortured and killed too slowly, when death was the only thing left to give release. But while it revealed the gruesome side of human existence, it also brought up many things good in human nature such as empathy, and many, very many of those who suffered the tortures of cancer in the breast, were heroines to their devastated friends.

NOTES

1 'One of the Most Grievous and Rebellious' Diseases: Defining, Diagnosing and the Causes of Cancers

1. D. Turner, *The Art of Surgery*, vol. 1 (London, 1722), p. 85. Turner had translated this from Latin: 'these Lines I met with in an antient Manuscript of Physic, placed under the Cancer. Si aliquem odis, / Ac infaelicem praecas: / Nec Pestis,/ Nec Lues,/ Nec Pandorae Pixis,/ Nec Podagra,/ Nec Calculus;/ His omnibus omissis,/ Si magis infaelicem,/ Habeat cancrum'.

2. In the order quoted: W. Nisbet, *An Inquiry into the History, Nature, Causes, and Different Modes of Treatment Hitherto Pursued, in the Cure of Scrophula and Cancer* (Edinburgh, 1795), p. 4; *The Modern Family Physician, or the Art of Healing Made Easy ... Extracted from ... Eminent Physical Writers* (London, 1775), p. 219; Pulteney cited in L. B. Coates, 'Female Disorders: Eighteenth-Century Medical Therapeutics in Britain and North America' (PhD dissertation, Birkbeck College, University of London, 2005), p. 64. Turner notes that it is 'the most deplorable of all others'. Turner, *The Art of Surgery*, vol. 1, p. 76. J. Ewart, *The History of Two Cases of Ulcerated Cancer of the Mamma* (Bath, 1794), p. v; also cited in Coates, 'Female Disorders', p. 64. For understanding early modern illness, A. Wear, *Knowledge and Practice in English Medicine, 1550–1680* (Cambridge: Cambridge University Press, 2000) and M. Stolberg, *Experiencing Illness and the Sick Body in Early Modern Europe* (Basingstoke and New York: Palgrave 2011) are essential reads.

3. Nisbet, *An Inquiry*, p. 4. For earlier similar thoughts, see also P. Dionis, *A Course of Chirurgical Operations, demonstrated in the royal garden at Paris*, 2nd edn (London, 1733), p. 247.

4. J. Aitken, *Principles of Midwifery, or Puerperal Medicine*, 2nd edn (Edinburgh, 1785), p. 122.

5. B. Bell, *A System of Surgery*, 6th edn, vol. 5 (Edinburgh, 1796), p. 170.

6. *A Compendium of Physic, and Surgery. For the Use of Young Practitioners* (London, 1769), p. 247.

7. H. Fearon, *A Treatise on Cancers; with an Account of a New and Successful Method of Operating, Particularly in Cancers of the Breast or Testis*, 3rd edn (London, 1790), pp. 6, 81–2.

8. T. Frewen, *Physiologia: or, The Doctrine of Nature, Comprehended in the Origin and Progression of Human Life; the Vital and Animal Functions; Diseases of Body and Mind* (London, 1780), p. 431.

9. B. Gooch, *The Chirurgical Works of Benjamin Gooch, Surgeon; a New Edn, with his Last Corrections and Additions*, vol. 3 (London, 1792), p. 174.

10. Society for Bettering the Condition and Increasing the Comforts of the Poor, *The Reports of the Society for Bettering the Condition and Increasing the Comforts of the Poor*, vol. 3 (London, 1798–1800), pp. 262–3.

11. L. Heister, *A General System of Surgery in Three Parts. Translated into English*, vol. 1 (London, 1743), p. 228.

12. See for example J. Guillemeau, *A Worthy Treatise of the Eyes Contayning the Knowledge and Cure of One Hundred and Thirtene Diseases, Incident vnto them... Set Forth by W. Bailey. D. of Phisick* (London, 1587), p. 62; J. J. Wecker, *A Compendious Chyrurgerie: Gathered, & Translated (especially) out of Wecker* (London, 1585), p. 106; P. Barrough, *The Methode of Phisicke Conteyning the Causes, Signes, and Cures of Inward Diseases in Mans Body from the Head to the Foote* (London, 1583), p. 274; Anon., *An Account of the Causes of Some Particular Rebellious Distempers Viz. the Scurvey, Cancers in Women's Breasts, &c.* ([London?], 1670), pp. 21, 24.

13. D. Turner, *The Art of Surgery: in which is Laid Down Such a General Idea of the Same ...*, vol. 1 (London, 1722), p. 76.

14. J. Astruc, *A Treatise on the Diseases of Women*, vol. 3 (London, 1767), p. 347–8.

15. J. Pearson, *Principles of Surgery, for the Use of Chirurgical Students* (London, 1788), p. 214.

16. J. Pearson, *Practical Observations on Cancerous Complaints* (London, 1793), pp. 3, 46–8. See also B. Peyrilhe, *A Dissertation on Cancerous Diseases* (London, 1777), p. 5; G. Wallis, *The Art of Preventing Diseases* (London, 1793), pp. 758–9; D. MacBride, *A Methodical Introduction to the Theory and Practice of Physic* (London, 1772), p. 625.

17. An example of a specific diagnosis is for example the diagnosis of Mrs Day's breast tumour as 'an imperfect schirrus of one Breast'. C. Bissett, Cases, Wellcome Library, MS 1964, p. 437. MacBride considered cancer and scrofula to be related. MacBride, *Methodical Introduction*, p. 625.

18. W. M., *The Queens Closet Opened, Incomparable Secrets in Physick, Chyrurgery, Preserving and Candying &c.* (London, 1659), p. 85.

19. B. Cornwell, *The Domestic Physician; or, Guardian of Health* (London, 1784), p. 523. Later he analyses the process further: 'The nipple sinks in, turgid veins are conspicuous, ramifying far about, and resembling a crab's claws', pp. 525–6. See also M. Flemyng, *An Introduction to Physiology* (London, 1759), p. 129. Similar teaching was given by a Gentleman of the Faculty in his *Every Lady Her Own Physician; or, The Closet Companion. Corrected and Revised by Silvester Mahon* (London, 1788), pp. 66–7; B. Gooch, *The Chirurgical Works of Benjamin Gooch, Surgeon; a New Edn, with his Last Corrections and Additions*, vol. 3 (London, 1792), pp. 176–7. On ancient Galenism, see V. Nutton, *Ancient Medicine* (London and New York: Routledge, 2004/7), especially pp. 230–47.

20. R. Guy, *Practical Observations on Cancers and Disorders of the Breast, Explaining their Different Appearances and Events. To which are Added, One Hundred Cases, Successfully Treated without Cutting* (London, [c. 1762]), p. 2. On the other hand there were the likes of John Burrows who wrote in the latter part of the eighteenth century on the characteristics of schirrus; in essence his understanding of the illness does not much differ from the definitions of cancer presented above. Burrows lists five special features which would make a schirrus: the presence of at least some hardness, insensibility, changes of colour only in an advanced state, formation by congestion, and the absence of abnormal heat. See J. Burrows, *A New Practical Essay on Cancers* (London, 1783), p. 35. Peyrilhe, who

considered, as mentioned above, that schirrus and cancer were different stages of the same disease, considered cancer to have several distinguishable stages. For him too the last stage was that of ulceration. Peyrilhe, *Dissertation on Cancerous Diseases*, pp. 5–9.

21. J. Warner, *Cases in Surgery; with Introductions, Operations and Remarks*, 4th edn (London, 1784), pp. 396–400.

22. R. Brookes, *The General Practice of Physic*, 2nd edn, vol. 2 (London, 1754), p. 121. Burrows stresses changes in painfulness, which increases greatly; the size of the tumour; the form of the tumour, which becomes more rugged; and changes in the skin. Burrows, *A New Practical Essay on Cancers*, pp. 51–2.

23. Gooch, *The Chirurgical Works*, vol. 3, p. 176.

24. Pliny, *The Historie of the World*, translated Into English by Philemon Holland Doctor of Physicke (London, 1634), sig. A3; Lanfranco of Milan, *Chirurgia Parua Lanfranci* (London, 1565), p. 20; Guillemeau, *A Worthy Treatise*, p. 39; J. Guillemeau, *A Treatise of One Hundred and Thirteene Diseases of the Eyes, and Eye-liddes* (London, 1622), sig. N12; Barrough, *The Methode of Phisicke*, p. 273; Wecker, *A Compendious Chyrurgerie*, p. 106; J. Banister, *The Workes of that Famous Chyrurgian, Mr. Iohn Banester by him Digested into Five Bookes* (London, 1633), pp. 58–9; R. Bayfield, *Enchiridion Medicum: Containing the Causes, Signs, and Cures of All those Diseases, that Do Chiefly Affect the Body of Man* (London, 1655), p. 292; P. Barbette, *Thesaurus Chirurgiae: The Chirurgical and Anatomical Works of Paul Barbette ...*, translated out of Low-Dutch into English (London, 1687), pp. 122–3. On eighteenth-century versions, see M. de la Vauguion, *A Compleat Body of Chirurgical Operations, Containing the Whole Practice of Surgery*, 2nd edn (London, 1707), pp. 87–8; R. Boulton, *A System of Rational and Practical Chirurgery* (London, 1713), p. 109; R. Wiseman, *Eight Chirurgical Treatises, ... in two volumes*, 6th edn, vol. 1 (London, 1734), p. 169; Brookes, *The General Practice of Physic*, p. 121; *A Compendium of Physic*, p. 247; W. Buchan, *Domestic Medicine: or, A Treatise on the Prevention and Cure of Diseases by Regimen and Simple Medicines*, 2nd edn (London, 1772), p. 601 (he speaks of the 'fancied resemblance' of the cancer roots to the crab); G. van Swieten, *An Abridgement of Baron Van Swieten's Commentaries upon the Aphorisms of the Celebrated Dr. Herman Boerhaave*, vol. 1 (London, 1773–5), p. 432; T. Marryat, *All the Prescriptions Contained in The New Practice of Physic, of Thomas Marryat, M.D. Translated into English by J. S. Dodd* (London, 1774), p. 135; Burrows, *A New Practical Essay on Cancers*, p. 52; Cornwell, *The Domestic Physician*, p. 523; N. Culpeper, *Culpeper's English Physician; and Complete Herbal* (London, 1789), p. 181; J. Latta, *A Practical System of Surgery*, vol. 2 (Edinburgh, 1793), p. 142; Wallis, *The Art of Preventing Diseases*, pp. 758–60.

25. S. Young, *Minutes of Cases of Cancer and Cancerous Tendency, Successfully Treated by Mr. Samuel Young, Surgeon* (London, 1815), p. 4. In 1800, Richard Nayler had written that the ancient metaphor of a crab was well suited to cancer because so little was known of the disease. What Young termed varicose veins, Nayler had termed 'hard chords'. R. Nayler, *A Cursory View of the Treatment of Ulcers, More Especially those of the Scrofulous, Phagedænic, & Cancerous Description* (Gloucester, 1800), pp. 130–1.

26. The pompion appears in L. Heister, *Medical, Chirurgical, and Anatomical Cases and Observations, translated from the German original by George Wirgman* (London, 1755), p. 605. Comparisons were habitually made to household items and foodstuffs. See Anon., *An Account*, p. 21; Wiseman, *Eight Chirurgical Treatises*, p. 169; Bayfield, *Enchiridion Medicum*, pp. 292–3; de la Vauguion, *A Compleat Body of Chirurgical Operations*, p. 88; W. Nisbet, *The Clinical Guide; or, A Concise View of the Leading Facts on the History, Nature, and Cure of Diseases; to which is Subjoined, a Practical Pharmacopoeia* (Edin-

burgh, 1793), p. 149; Pearson, *Practical Observations*, pp. 42–3; J. Parkinson, *Medical Admonitions Addressed to Families, Respecting the Practice of Domestic Medicine, and the Preservation of Health*, 3rd edn, vol. 2 (London, 1799), pp. 467–9. Tissot mentions a nut as the smallest size. S. A. D. Tissot, *The Lady's Physician. A Practical Treatise on the Various Disorders Incident to the Fair Sex, Translated by an Eminent Physician* (London, 1766), p. 42. Melmoth Guy talks about the sizes of tumours as for example a pea, a walnut (in four cases), a large orange, a pint bason, a common tea-cup, a pigeon's egg, a large golden-pippin, a hen's egg, a China orange and a French roll (extended from the clavicle to the axilla). See M. Guy, *A Select Number of Schirrhus and Cancerous Cases Successfully Treated Without Cutting, by the Peculiar Remedy of Melmoth Guy* (London, 1777), pp. 3, 6, 14, 18, 22, 24, 25, 29, 31, 35, 36, 39.

27. Wecker, *A Compendious Chyrurgerie*, p. 107; Banister, *The Workes*, p. 59; Anon., *An Account*, pp. 21, 23; E. Maynwaringe, *The Frequent, but Unsuspected Progress of Pains, Inflammations, Tumors, Apostems, Ulcers, Cancers, Gangrenes, and Mortifications Internal Therein* (London, 1679); R. Guy, *An Essay on Scirrhous Tumours, and Cancers* (London, 1759), pp. 36, 47; Buchan, *Domestic Medicine*, p. 600; W. Fordyce, *Fragmenta Chirurgica & Medica* (London, 1784), pp. 17–18.

28. Pearson, *Principles of Surgery*, pp. 216–7.

29. H. J. G. Bloom, W. W. Richardson, E. J. Harries, 'Natural History of Untreated Breast Cancer (1805–1933). Comparison of Untreated and Treated Cases According to Histological Grade of Malignancy', *British Medical Journal*, 5299: July (1962), pp. 213–21, on p. 215.

30. Cornwell, *The Domestic Physician*, p. 527. See also Astruc, *A Treatise on the Diseases of Women*, vol. 3, pp. 352–3; Gooch, *The Chirurgical Works*, vol. 3, pp. 179–80, 182.

31. Brookes, *The General Practice of Physic*, pp. 121–2. Others used very similar imagery. See Turner, *The Art of Surgery*, vol. 1 p. 77; Buchan, *Domestic Medicine*, pp. 601–2; Burrows, *A New Practical Essay on Cancers*, pp. 52–3; Culpeper, *Culpeper's English Physician*, p. 181; R. White, *Practical Surgery: Containing the Description, Causes, and Treatment of Each Complaint; Together with the Most Approved Methods of Operating*, 2nd edn (London, 1796), p. 43.

32. Anon., *An Account*, pp. 21, 25; Turner, *The Art of Surgery*, vol. 1, p. 81.

33. Nisbet, *An Inquiry*, pp. 159–60. See also Pearson, *Principles of Surgery*, pp. 217–8.

34. Bloom, Richardson and Harries, 'Natural History of Untreated Breast Cancer', p. 220.

35. B. Duden, *The Woman Beneath the Skin. A Doctor's Patients in Eighteenth-Century Germany* (Cambridge, MA and London: Harvard University Press, 1991/7), p. 15; Wear, *Knowledge and Practice*, p. 255. On early modern hierarchies of the senses, see S. Clark, *Vanities of the Eye. Vision in Early Modern European Culture* (Oxford: Oxford University Press, 2007), pp. 9–13, 20–1. See also S. Biernoff, *Sight and Embodiment in the Middle Ages. Ocular Desires* (Basingstoke: Palgrave, 2002), pp. 1–2.

36. Daniel Turner wrote that he had tasted the sand-like salt excreted by a patient who had died of cancer. He emphasized that he had rinsed the salt several times before the experiment. Turner, *The Art of Surgery*, vol. 1, p. 87. On premodern attitudes to the bodily fluids, see for example J. R. Gillis, 'From Ritual to Romance: Toward and Alternative History of Love', in C. Z. Stearns and P. N. Stearns (eds) *Emotion and Social Change. Toward a New Psychohistory* (New York and London: Holmes & Meier, 1988), pp. 87–121; and on the importance of bowel movement, R. Porter and D. Porter, *In Sickness and in Health. The British Experience 1650–1850* (London: Fourth Estate, 1988), p. 50.

37. Account of a tumour in breast, British Library (hereafter BL), Sloane MS 4078, f. 114.

38. Morgan, Casebook, 1714–1747, Wellcome Library (hereafter Wellcome) MS 3631, f. 63.
39. J. Hunter, *The Case Books of John Hunter FRS*, ed. E. Allen, J. L. Turk and Sir R. Murley (London: Royal Society of Medicine Services, 1993), p. 57 (italics mine). On the life of John Hunter, see W. Moore, *The Knife Man. Blood, Body-Snatching and the Birth of Modern Surgery* (London: Bantam, 2005); on cancer p. 337.
40. Wiseman, *Eight Chirurgical Treatises*, p. 168.
41. Duden, *The Woman Beneath the Skin*, pp. 85, 86–7. See also M. Yalom, *A History of the Breast* (London: HarperCollins, 1997), p. 219.
42. Duden, *The Woman Beneath the Skin*, pp. 180–1.
43. Anon., *An Account*, p. 29.
44. Astruc, *A Treatise on the Diseases of Women*, vol. 3, pp. 354–5, 356.
45. One example: H-F. Le Dran, *The Operations in Surgery of Mons. Le Dran ... translated by Mr. Gataker*, 3rd edn (London, 1757), p. 287.
46. Lanfranco, *Chirurgia Parua Lanfranci*, p. 19; Guillemeau, *A Worthy Treatise*, p. 41; Guillemeau, *A Treatise*, sig. O1; Nutton, *Ancient Medicine*, pp. 23, 35.
47. Guillemeau, *A Worthy Treatise*, pp. 41–2; Guillemeau, *A Treatise*, sig. O1–O1v; *Maynwaringe, The Frequent, but Unsuspected Progress of Pains*, pp. 194–5; Frewen, *Physiologia*, p. 431.
48. Banister, *The Workes*, p. 59.
49. Lanfranco, *Chirurgia Parua Lanfranci*, p. 20; Banister, *The Workes*, p. 59.
50. D. Irish, *Levamen Infirmi: or, Cordial Counsel to the Sick and Diseased* (Guilford, 1700), pp. 19–20.
51. J. Moyle, John. *The Experienced Chirurgion* (London, 1703), p. 48. See also Turner, *The Art of Surgery*, vol. 1, p. 4.
52. Boulton, *A System of Rational and Practical Chirurgery*, p. 109.
53. S. Partlicius, *A New Method of Physick: or, A Short View of Paracelsus and Galen's Practice* (London, 1654), p. 481. On melancholy as an early modern disease, see for example M. S. Sánchez, 'Melancholy and Female Illness: Habsburg Women and Politics at the Court of Philip III', *Journal of Women's History*, 8:2 (1996), pp. 81–102; H. Mikkeli, 'A Melancholy Man – Between a Medical Discourse and a Literary Topos', in M. Kaartinen and A. Korhonen (eds), *Bodies in Evidence. Perspectives on the History of the Body in Early Modern Europe* (Turku: Cultural History, University of Turku, Turku, 1997), pp. 13–40; Clark, *Vanities of the Eye*, pp. 50–2.
54. D. de Moulin, *A Short History of Breast Cancer* (Dordrecht, Boston, MA and London: Kluwer Academic Publishers, 193/1989), pp. 22–3. Peyrilhe, *Dissertation on Cancerous Diseases*, p. 14, wondered about the causes 'of so great a metamorphosis' that turned the lymph cancerous.
55. Anon., *An Account*, p. 20.
56. *Bibliotheca Anatomica, Medica, Chirurgica, &c. Containing a Description of the Several Parts of the Body: Each Done by Some One or More Eminent Physician or Chirurgeon; with their Diseases and Cures*, vol. 1 (London, 1711–14), p. 83. Many authors reiterated that of all its seats, cancer was most frequent in the breasts of women.
57. Cornwell, *The Domestic Physician*, p. 523. See also K. Nolte, '*Carcinoma Uteri* and "Sexual Debauchery" – Morality, Cancer and Gender in the Nineteenth Century', *Social History of Medicine*, 21:1 (2008), pp. 31–46.
58. Gooch, *The Chirurgical Works*, vol. 3, p. 178; Tissot, *The Lady's Physician*, p. 41; H. Smith, 'Gynecology and Ideology in Seventeenth-Century England', in B. A. Carroll

(ed.), *Liberating Women's History. Theoretical and Critical Essays* (Urbana, Chicago, IL and London: University of Illinois Press, 1976), pp. 97–114.

59. See also E. Shorter, *Women's Bodies. A Social History of Women's Encounter with Health, Ill-Health, and Medicine* (New Brunswick and London: Transaction, 1991/7), p. 243.

60. W. Charleton, *Natural History of Nutrition, Life, and Vol.untary Motion Containing All the New Discoveries of Anatomist's and Most Probable Opinions of Physicians* (London, 1659), p. 31.

61. Private autopsies took place every now and then with the consent of the relatives. Official anatomy-school autopsies could be carried out only on the legally obtained bodies of criminals after execution. The Anatomy Act of 1832 made it possible for dead bodies in general to be part of 'medical trade'. R. McGrath, *Seeing Her Sex. Medical Archives and the Female Body* (Manchester and New York: Manchester University Press, 2002), p. 63; on late medieval Italian dissections, see K. Park, *Secrets of Women. Gender, Generation, and the Origins of Human Dissection* (New York: Zone), especially pp. 121–31.

62. J. Ward, *Diary of the Rev. John Ward, A.M., Vicar of Stratford-Upon-Avon, Extending from 1648 to 1679. From the Original MSS Preserved in the Library of the Medical Society of London. Arranged by Charles Severn, M.D.* (London, 1839), p. 247. Also cited in de Moulin, *A Short History of Breast Cancer*, p. 27. Payne also discusses Mrs Townshend's case, see L. Payne, *With Words and Knives. Learning Medical Dispassion in Early Modern England* (Aldershot and Burlington, VT: Ashgate, 2007), pp. 71–3.

63. Anon., *An Account*, p. 23; A. Read, *The Manuall of the Anatomy or Dissection of the Body of Man Containing the Enumeration, and Description of the Parts of the Same, Which Usually Are Shewed in the Publike Anatomicall Exercises* (London, 1638), pp. 276–7.

64. H. King, *Hippocrates' Woman. Reading the Female Body in Ancient Greece* (London and New York: Routledge, 1998), p. 28. Breasts and the womb, of course, were also connected with each other. See also pp. 34–5, where King notes for example that the paleness of the nipples could reveal a disease of the womb. On late medieval thoughts on the uterus, see Park, *Secrets of Women*, pp. 103–120.

65. King, *Hippocrates' Woman*, p. 28.

66. Read, *The Manuall*, p. 282.

67. Charleton, *Natural History of Nutrition*, pp. 29–30.

68. Ibid., p. 31.

69. J. Ball, *The Female Physician: or, Every Woman Her Own Doctress* (London, 1770), p. 85. Benjamin Bell also considered women's breasts as the most frequent seat of cancer. Bell, *A System of Surgery*, vol. 5, p. 169. He too thought this was due to their glandulous nature. Ibid, p. 170.

70. Fearon, *A Treatise on Cancers*, p. 35.

71. *Modern Family Physician*, p. 219.

72. Fearon, *A Treatise on Cancers*, p. 35. White first noted that the lips and breasts were the most prone to cancer. White, *Practical Surgery*, p. 42, but later noted that schirri and cancer 'chiefly affect the breasts of women'. Ibid., p. 367.

73. Guy, *An Essay*, 1759, 5; Guy, *Practical Observations*, p. 9. On the dangers of these glandules, see Anon., *An Account*, p. 21; Nisbet, *The Clinical Guide*, p. 149; Nisbet, *An Inquiry*, pp. 131–2; Moyle, *The Experienced Chirurgion*, p. 48; Burrows, *A New Practical Essay on Cancers*, p. 35; Latta, *A Practical System of Surgery*, vol. 2, pp. 509–10; *The Edinburgh Practice of Physic and Surgery* (London, 1800), p. 681. Peyrilhe considered the proximity of the heart to be the key to the risks of the breasts. Peyrilhe, *Dissertation on Cancerous Diseases*, pp. 9–10. In vitalistic terms, Richard Carmichael concluded that female breasts were 'so often

the seat of Carcinoma' because they had so few arteries; there was not much circulation, and as there was so many lymphatics, their vital powers were dangerously low. R. Carmichael, *An Essay on the Effects of Carbonate of Iron, upon Cancer, with an Inquiry into the Nature of that Disease* (Dublin and London, 1806), pp. 59–60.

74. Astruc, *A Treatise on the Diseases of Women*, vol. 3, p. 283. The lymphatic importance of male and female breasts is repeated on pp. 286–7.

75. Read, *The Manuall of the Anatomy*, p. 273; *Medical Commentaries ... Exhibiting a Concise View of the Latest and Most Important Discoveries in Medicine and Medical Philosophy. Collected and Published by Andrew Duncan*, vol. 9 (Edinburgh, 1795), pp. 197–200. Duden, *The Woman Beneath the Skin*, p. 117. Breasts return us to the question of Laqueur and his one sex model. T. Laqueur, *Making Sex: Body and Gender from the Greeks to Freud* (Cambridge, MA: Harvard University Press, 1992), esp. p. 8; M. E. Fissell, *Vernacular Bodies. The Politics of Reproduction in Early Modern England* (Oxford and New York: Oxford University Press, 2004), pp. 12–13. On the breast and Laqueur, see S. Richter, *Missing the Breast. Gender, Fantasy, and the Body in the German Enlightenment* (Seattle and London: University of Washington Press, 2006), pp. 81–2. Richter names Londa Schiebinger as an exemplary model against Laqueur: L. Schiebinger, *Nature's Body. Gender in the Making of Modern Science* (Boston, MA: Beacon Press, 1993). See also M. Baker, 'Feminist Post-Structuralist Engagements with History', *Rethinking History*, 2:3 (1998), pp. 371–8. Today the case against the one-sex model of Thomas Lacqueur is strong; most scholars agree that differences between male and female patients were considered significant enough to differentiate for example treatment. See W. D. Churchill, 'The Medical Practice of the Sexed Body: Women, Men, and Disease in Britain, *Circa* 1600–1740', *Social History of Medicine*, 18:1 (2005), pp. 3–22, see esp. p. 10. On the two-sex model in antiquity, see King, *Hippocrates' Woman*, pp. 7, 11–12, 27, who argues for a multitude of understandings of the sexes. On early modern thought, H. King, *Midwifery, Obstetrics and the Rise of Gynaecology: The Uses of a Sixteenth-Century Compendium* (Aldershot: Ashgate Publishing, 2007), especially pp. 13–14, 23, 26–7.

76. It was possible to conceive that men could menstruate regularly – from their fingertips, from varicose veins, or indeed through the penis. See Duden, *The Woman Beneath the Skin*, pp. 116–7. An English case: A menstruating man in his early twenties, William Calloway from Cornwall, had had his bleedings for several years. A surgeon, William Hamley, mentioned to John Hunter that William Calloway had 'regular Menstrual Discharge of Blood from the Urethra (ritu Mulierum) which continued on him for two or three days'. This note is included in Hunter, *The Case Books*, p. 188.

77. Le Dran, *The Operations in Surgery*, p. 292; Heister, *A General System of Surgery*, vol. 1, p. 229.

78. Bayfield, *Enchiridion Medicum*, pp. 293–4.

79. Guy, *An Essay*, pp. 58–9.

80. Guy, *A Select Number of Schirrhus and Cancerous Cases*, pp. 9–10. It is possible that Melmoth Guy used the same 'Plunkett's Pultice' used by Richard Guy. I assume that Richard was his father, as he refers to his father's patients, and mentions that his father used the same cure. Richard Guy mentions that Plunkett and his predecessors had successfully used the poultice for a hundred years. Guy, *An Essay*, passim. In Guy, *Practical Observations*, pp. xv–xvi, he wrote that there had been rumours that he used caustics, but he denied this, assuring readers that it was indeed a poultice, not caustics, that he used, and caused hardly any pain. *The London Practice of Physic. For the Use of Physicians and Younger Practitioners. Wherein the Definition and Symptoms of Diseases are Laid Down,*

and the Present Method of Cure (London, 1769), pp. 183–4, however, revealed the ingredients of this famous poultice, and they included white arsenic. The pain caused may have been numbed by the opiates included in the poultice. The recipe was also printed in MacBride, *Methodical Introduction*, p. 626. Nisbet too lists it in a group with escharotics using arsenic or mercury. Comments also in Nisbet, *The Clinical Guide*, p. 151; J. Townsend, *A Guide to Health; being Cautions and Directions in the Treatment of Diseases. Designed Chiefly for the Use of Students*, 2nd edn, vol. 2 (London, 1795–96), p. 464; R. J. Thornton, *The Philosophy of Medicine: or, Medical Extracts on the Nature of Health and Disease, including the Laws of the Animal Œconomy, and the Doctrines of Pneumatic Medicine*, vol. 5, 4th edn (London, 1800), p. 414.

81. Guy, *A Select Number of Schirrhus and Cancerous Cases*, p. 38.
82. B. di Dominiceti, *Medical Anecdotes of the Last Thirty Years, Illustrated with Medical Truths, and Addressed to the Medical Faculty; but in an Especial Manner, to the People at Large* (London, 1781), p. 376.
83. Ibid., pp. 376–7.
84. Ibid., pp. 377.
85. For medieval ideas on the menses, see M. Green (ed.), *The Trotula. An English Translation of the Medieval Compendium of Women's Medicine* (Philadelphia, PA: University of Pennsylvania Press, 2002), pp. 66–71. Patricia Crawford has noted that 'women regarded the absence of menstruation as a symptom requiring treatment', P. Crawford, 'Attitudes to Menstruation in Seventeenth-Century England', *Past & Present*, 91 (1981), pp. 47–73; King, *Midwifery*, pp. 52–9.
86. Anon., *An Account*, p. 22; de Moulin, *A Short History of Breast Cancer*, p. 2; King, *Hippocrates' Woman*, pp. 28–9; Nutton, *Ancient Medicine*, pp. 23, 79; Churchill, 'The Medical Practice of the Sexed Body', pp. 20.
87. Wecker, *A Compendious Chyrurgerie*, p. 106; S. A. D. Tissot, *Advice to People in General, with Respect to their Health. Translated from the French edn of Dr. Tissot's Avis au People ... in Two Volumes*, 5th edn, vol. 2 (Dublin, 1769), p. 217; Van Swieten, *An Abridgement*, p. 434; James Latta suggested that the most dangerous age was between 36 and 48, Latta, *A Practical System of Surgery*, vol. 1, p. 144; Townsend, *A Guide to Health*, p. 462.
88. Maynwaringe, *The Frequent, but Unsuspected Progress of Pains*, p. 195. See also Guy, *An Essay*, p. 64–5; Nutton, *Ancient Medicine*, p. 30.
89. Dionis, *A Course of Chirurgical Operations*, p. 249. Supported by W. Norford, *An Essay on the General Method of Treating Cancerous Tumors* (London, 1753), p. 63; Nisbet, *An Inquiry*, pp. 185–6.
90. Latta, *A Practical System of Surgery*, vol. 2, pp. 509–10.
91. Fearon, *A Treatise on Cancers*, p. 31; for more on his views on this question, see pp. 42–4, and for a case of schirrus which healed after the patient's menses returned, pp. 64–5.
92. J. Hill, *Plain and Useful Directions for those who are Afflicted with Cancers*, 2nd edn (London, [c. 1773]), p. 22. See also. F. Home, *Principia medicinae*, 4 edn (Edinburgh, 1770), pp. 220–1.
93. Pearson, *Principles of Surgery*, p. 211. See also Peyrilhe, *Dissertation on Cancerous Diseases*, p. 11.
94. Tissot, *Advice to People in General*, p. 220.
95. Guy, *An Essay*, pp. 64–5.
96. Nayler, *A Cursory View of the Treatment of Ulcers*, p. 136.

97. De Moulin, *A Short History of Breast Cancer*, p. 37. The wealth of my source material supports this notion. Many supported this idea, even though they admitted that cancer could trouble younger people as well. Heister, *A General System of Surgery*, vol. 1, p. 229.

98. Carmichael, *An Essay*, p. 59. Nutton, *Ancient Medicine*, p. 23.

99. Carmichael, *An Essay*, p. 59.

100. Buchan, *Domestic Medicine*, p. 600; Pearson, *Principles of Surgery*, p. 209.

101. Guy, *Practical Observations*, pp. 8–9.

102. Ibid., p. 9.

103. J. S., *Paidon Nosemata· = or Childrens Diseases Both Outward and Inward* (London, 1664), p. 22.

104. Cornwell, *The Domestic Physician*, p. 524.

105. Perry, 'Colonizing the Breast', p. 214.

106. Paré cited in Yalom, *History of the Breast*, p. 71.

107. King, *Midwifery*, p. 24.

108. Shorter, *Women's Bodies*, p. 244.

109. On the meanings of breastfeeding in the seventeenth century, see G. K. Paster, *The Body Embarrassed. Drama and the Disciplines of Shame in Early Modern England* (Ithaca, NY: Cornell University Press, 1993), pp. 197–208, 215–80. On the political breast in the eighteenth century, see R. Perry, 'Colonizing the Breast: Sexuality and Maternity in Eighteenth-Century England', *Journal of the History of Sexuality*, 2:2 (1991), pp. 204–34. On the polemics, S. Richter, *Missing the Breast. Gender, Fantasy, and the Body in the German Enlightenment* (Seattle and London: University of Washington Press, 2006), pp. 12–13, 84–5. See also V. Lastinger, 'Re-Defining Motherhood: Breast-Feeding and the French Enlightenment', *Women's Studies*, 25:6 (1996), pp. 603–17. On the new woman in the ideal family of the French Revolution, see L. Hunt, *Family Romance of the French Revolution* (Berkeley and Los Angeles, CA: University of California Press, 1992), pp. 156–60; on Mercier, see R. Forsström, *Possible Worlds. The Idea of Happiness in the Utopian Vision of Louis-Sébastien Mercier* (Helsinki: SKS, 2002), pp. 140–52.

110. W. Rowley, *A Practical Treatise on Diseases of the Breasts of Women. Containing Directions for the Proper Management of Breasts during Lying-in, with Observations on the Present Defective Methods of Practice* (London, 1772), pp. iii, viii, 43; W. Rowley, *A Treatise on the Management of Female Breasts During Childbed; and Several New Observations on Cancerous Diseases*, 2nd edn (London, 1790), pp. 4–5, 21.

111. Rowley, *Practical Treatise*, p. 22.

112. 'Journal', *Sun*, 28 Aug 28, 1768, in Lady M. Coke, *The Letters and Journals of Lady Mary Coke, vol. first, 1756–1767* (Bath: Privately printed, Kingsmead reprints, 1970), p. 348.

113. Young, *Minutes*, p. 66. There was probably good news about this case. Her treatments came to a halt when it was discovered that she was pregnant, and Dr Young noted months later that he had not heard from her since – she had been asked to return if there was pain. Ibid., pp. 74, 75.

114. In the sixteenth century, the German surgeon Wilhem Fabry held such an opinion. De Moulin, *A Short History of Breast Cancer*, p. 18.

115. J. L. Epstein, 'Writing the Unspeakable: Fanny Burney's Mastectomy and the Fictive Body', *Representations*, 16 (1986), pp. 131–166.

116. F. Burney, *The Journals and Letters of Fanny Burney (Madame D'Arblay), vol. 6, France 1803–1812* (Oxford: Clarendon Press, 1975), pp. 475, 563.

117. Banister, *The Workes*, pp. 131–2. With examples: *Medical Commentaries*, vol. 9, pp. 197–200. It was noted in it that '[w]hen milk tumours and indurations suppurate, they

often occasion obstinate and painful ulcers, which not unfrequently acquire a truly bad aspect'. Ibid., p. 199.

118. Astruc, *A Treatise on the Diseases of Women*, vol. 3, pp. 348–9. This idea easily led to a diagnosis of such formations as cancerous, and many physicians and surgeons were concerned about quacks who claimed to cure cancers even though what they were curing were milk abscesses. Parkinson, *Medical Admonitions*, pp. 472–3.

119. Astruc, *A Treatise on the Diseases of Women*, vol. 3, p. 350.

120. Bell, *A System of Surgery*, vol. 1, pp. 144–5. Of similar mind were Guy, *Practical Observations*, pp. 10–11; Tissot, *Advice to People in General*, p. 225, who wrote that milk abscesses had to be dissolved immediately.

121. Bell, *A System of Surgery*, vol. 1, pp. 145–7.

122. Burrows, *A New Practical Essay on Cancers*, pp. 41–2.

123. Nayler, *A Cursory View of the Treatment of Ulcers*, p. 135. This was in accordance with for example what Nisbet had written earlier – he considered barrenness and refusal to breastfeed the greatest risk factors for women. Nisbet, *An Inquiry*, p. 132. Not many voices were heard saying that suckling and cancer had nothing to do with each other. Daniel Turner (1722) was exceptional in noting that 'I could not say that I ever knew a Tumour from Milk, degenerating into that Disease'. Turner, *The Art of Surgery*, vol. 1, p. 74. Henry Fearon quite radically attested that milk abscesses did not have a tendency to turn cancerous, and that in fact he had never seen such a case. Fearon, *A Treatise on Cancers*, p. 25.

124. Hippocrates's *Maladies*, cited in L. S. Dixon, *Perilous Chastity. Women and Illness in Pre-Enlightenment Art and Medicine* (Ithaca, NY and London: Cornell University Press, 1995), p. 17.

125. De Moulin, *A Short History of Breast Cancer*, p. 38.

126. Heister, *A General System of Surgery*, vol. 1, p. 229.

127. Dionis, *A Course of Chirurgical Operations*, p. 249.

128. Gooch, *The Chirurgical Works*, vol. 3, p. 184; Buchan, *Domestic Medicine*, p. 600.

129. Cornwell, *The Domestic Physician*, pp. 523–4, 525.

130. J. Nooth, *Observations on the Treatment of Scirrhous Tumours of the Breast to which is Added a New and Efficacious Mode of Treating the Ulcerated Cancer*, 2nd edn (London, 1806), p. 5.

131. De Moulin, *A Short History of Breast Cancer*, p. 34.

132. Fearon, *A Treatise on Cancers*, pp. 26–7, 30–1. Perhaps such a natural disposition was the cause of the death from breast cancer of Margaret Banyard (née Cutting) from Wickham Market in Suffolk. She had apparently lost most of her tongue when she was four years old to what was considered cancer. She had retained her ability to speak, but was considered such a curiosity that as a young woman she had been examined by the Royal Society. She died in August 1773 when she was fifty-three. J. Morley, *The Eighteenth Edn, Eevised, of an Essay, on the Nature and Cure of Schrophulous Disorders, Commonly Called the King's Evil; Deduced from Long Observation and Practice* (London, 1778), pp. 67–9.

133. Dr Willis considered even a minor blow enough to cause the nervous liquid to form a tumour in women's breasts. T. Willis, *Dr. Willis's Practice of Physick* (London, 1684), p. 202.

134. See for example Norford, *An Essay*, pp. 66–7. For cases and further discussion, see M. Kaartinen, 'Making Sense of Illness. Gendering Breast Cancer in the Eighteenth Century', in Jörg Rogge et al. (eds) *Making Sense in History* (Mainz: Transcript, 2013 forthcoming).

135. De Moulin, *A Short History of Breast Cancer*, p. 34.

136. Wiseman, *Eight Chirurgical Treatises*, p. 167, other cases noting the same advice: pp. 175, 183.

137. Buchan, *Domestic Medicine*, pp. 601, 606. Similar terms in Culpeper, *Culpeper's English Physician*, pp. 181, 183; L. Mansey, *The Practical Physician; or, Medical Instructor. Pointing Out Remedies for the Various Diseases of Mankind* (London, 1800), p. 375. See also Arscott Family Physical Receipts, Wellcome MS 981, ff. 160–1; D. Turner, *De Morbis Cutaneis. A Treatise of Diseases Incident to the Skin* (London, 1714), p. 76; Home, *Principia medicinae*, p. 220, warned against outward friction.

138. Hill, *Plain and Useful Directions*, p. 7.

139. A. F. M. Willich, *Lectures on Diet and Regimen: Being a Systematic Inquiry into the Most Rational Means of Preserving Health and Prolonging Life* (London, 1800), pp. 277–8.

140. She was the daughter-in-law of a West-India merchant, Jonathan Ewer, esquire. Guy, *An Essay*, p. 79–81.

141. J. L. Vives, *The Passions of the Soul. The Third Book of* De Anima et Vita. trans. C. G. Noreña (Lewiston, Queenston, Lampeter: Edwin Mellen Press, 1990), p. 96; Hippocrates, *Hippocrates's Treatise on the Preservation of Health* (London, 1776), pp. 38, 68; de Moulin, *A Short History of Breast Cancer*, p. 24, 37. See also S. Knuuttila, *Emotions, in Ancient and Medieval Philosophy* (Oxford: Oxford University Press, 2006); F. B. Alberti, 'Emotions in the Early Modern Medical Tradition', in F. B. Alberti (ed.), *Medicine, Emotion and Disease, 1700–1950* (Basingstoke and New York: Palgrave, 2006), pp. 1–21. Considering passions to cause diseases such as cancers is not far from the modern idea that a woman causes her breast cancer by her own thoughts and actions: she works too hard, worries too much, suffers excessively from the adversities of life such as divorce or a death in the family, and so on. Paradoxically, this psychoanalytical discourse suggests that one should be able to heal oneself by changing these psychological patterns. M. Laiho, Sairaskuva – sairaan kuva – sairas kuva, in M. Laiho and I. Ruoho (eds), *Median merkitsemät. Ruumis ja sukupuoli kuvassa* (Jyväskylä: PS-kustannus, 2005), pp. 69–101.

142. Wiseman, *Eight Chirurgical Treatises*, p. 167.

143. Cornwell, *The Domestic Physician*, p. 525.

144. W. Falconer, *A Dissertation on the Influence of the Passions upon Disorders of the Body* (London, 1788), p. xiii.

145. Grief had many intensities. Walter Charleton listed the following: 'Discontent, Sollicitude, Vexation, Sadness, Sorrow, Affliction, Misery, Lamentation, Weeping and Howling'. W. Charleton, *A Natural History of the Passions*, 2nd edn (London, 1701), p. 128.

146. Willich, *Lectures*, p. 570. See also Nisbet, *An Inquiry*, p. 186; S. H. Mendelson, *The Mental World of Stuart Women. Three Studies* (Brighton: Harvester, 1987), p. 111; L. M. Beier, *Sufferers & Healers. The Experience of Illness in Seventeenth-Century England* (London and New York: Routledge, 1987), p. 236; Porter and Porter, *In Sickness and in Health*, p. 64; J. Eilola, "Ehkä se on Jumalasta, mutta voi se olla pahoista ihmisistäkin ...' Sairauden kokeminen, tulkinta ja parantaminen uuden ajan alussa', in H. Roiko-Jokela (ed.), *Vanhuus, vaivat erilaiset* (Jyväskylä: Jyväskylän Historiallinen Yhdistys, 1999), pp. 95–144; J. Sarjala, *Music, Morals, and the Body. An Academic Issue in Turku, 1653–1808* (Helsinki: SKS, 2001), p. 132.

147. Willich, *Lectures*, pp. 571–2. On these dangers, see also Charleton, *Natural History of the Passions*, pp. 150–2; Falconer, *Dissertation*, pp. xiv, 17–18.

148. Buchan, *Domestic Medicine*, p. 600.

149. Fearon, *A Treatise on Cancers*, p. 31.

150. J. Rodman, *A Practical Explanation of Cancer in the Female Breast, with the Method of Cure, and Cases of Illustration* (Paisley, 1815), passim.

151. This example was Miss A—y, who was the granddaughter of the 'Earl of H—t'. Guy, *Practical Observations*, p. 73.

152. Peyrilhe, *Dissertation on Cancerous Diseases*, p. 43. See also de Moulin, *A Short History of Breast Cancer*, p. 38; Coates, 'Female Disorders', p. 61.

153. Buchan, *Domestic Medicine*, 1772, p. 601.

154. Bissett, Cases, Wellcome MS 1964, ff. 435–436.

155. Society of Physicians in London, *Medical Observations and Inquiries*, 2nd edn, vol. 4 (London, 1772), p. 358.

156. Fearon, *A Treatise on Cancers*, p. 32.

157. Nisbet, *The Clinical Guide*, p. 150.

158. Pearson, *Principles of Surgery*, p. 209.

159. W. Rowley, *Seventy Four Select Cases, with the Manner of Cure, and the Preparation of the Remedies* (London, 1779), p. 10.

160. Robert John Thornton expressly did not believe cancer contagious. Thornton, *The Philosophy of Medicine*, vol. 5, p. 411.

161. Peyrilhe, *Dissertation on Cancerous Diseases*, pp. 45–6.

162. Ibid., p. 46.

163. De Moulin, *A Short History of Breast Cancer*, p. 24.

164. D. Nirenberg, *Communities of Violence. Persecution of Minorities in the Middle Ages* (Princeton, NJ: Princeton University Press, 1996), p. 57, and more on leprosy pp. 95–6.

165. De Moulin, *A Short History of Breast Cancer*, p. 24.

166. Mentioned in passing for example in Cornwell, *The Domestic Physician*, p. 525. Richard Guy mentions that Tulpius has strong proof of the contagious nature of cancer, but Guy merely reiterates British examples and two foreign lesser known examples. Guy, *An Essay*, p. 62–3. Lorenz Heister, for many a great German authority on cancers, posited that there was no foundation for this idea. Heister, *A General System of Surgery*, vol. 1, p. 230. Peyrilhe notes Tulpius's other case, in which a husband tried to suck out his wife's cancer, with the sad result that both of them ended up dead. His cancer took seat in his jaw. Peyrilhe, *Dissertation on Cancerous Diseases*, pp. 43–4.

167. Pearson, *Practical Observations*, pp. 22–3.

168. Anon., *An Account*, passim; W. Beckett, *New Discoveries relating to the Cure of Cancers*, 2nd edn (London, 1712); Guy, *An Essay*, p. 63; Peyrilhe, *Dissertation on Cancerous Diseases*, p. 44; Pearson, *Practical Observations*, pp. 24–5 is critical but Pearson, *Principles of Surgery*, p. 222 had noted in passing that 'An insupportable and fatal nausea has been the consequence of imprudently tasting it'.

169. Anon., *An Account*, pp. 24–5.

170. Willis, *Dr. Willis's Practice of Physick*, p. 202.

171. Latta, *A Practical System of Surgery*, vol. 1, p. 144.

172. Beckett, *New Discoveries*, p. 37.

173. Ibid., p. 36.

174. Ibid., p. 37.

175. Ibid., pp. 36–7. On early modern medicine and the relationship to the natural world, see M. Pelling, *The Common Lot. Sickness, Medical Occupations and the Urban Poor in Early Modern England* (London and New York: Longman, 1998), pp. 19–37.

176. Beckett, *New Discoveries*, pp. 42–3.

177. Ibid., p. 40. Guy, *An Essay*, p. 62, refers to this case.

178. Beckett, *New Discoveries*, p. 42–3. Also in Guy, *An Essay*, pp. 62–3.
179. Latta, *A Practical System of Surgery*, vol. 1, p. 140.
180. Pearson, *Practical Observations*, pp. 25–6.
181. B. Gooch, *Cases and Practical Remarks in Surgery. With Sketches of Machines, of Simple Construction, Easy Application, and Approved Use* (London, 1758), pp. 39–40. Retold in his later work, Gooch, *The Chirurgical Works*, vol. 2, p.127.

2 'But Sad Resources': Treating Cancer in the Eighteenth Century

1. Astruc, *A Treatise on the Diseases of Women*, vol. 3, p. 355; Burrows, *A New Practical Essay on Cancers*, pp. 57–8. Le Dran added to these difficulties another challenge: he stated that because all cancers were different, they should be treated differently. Le Dran, *The Operations in Surgery*, p. 292–3.
2. Astruc, *A Treatise on the Diseases of Women*, vol. 3, p. 355.
3. This was again ancient wisdom, Nutton, *Ancient Medicine*, p. 173.
4. Patients feared surgical operations greatly. I return to this topic in detail below.
5. The roots of this process can be found in sixteenth-century developments in anatomy. For example Vesalius urged physicians to return to the ideal medicine of Hippocrates and Galen and work with their hands, rather than leaving that to surgeons. Park, *Secrets of Women*, p. 244.
6. See for example Wecker, *A Compendious Chyrurgerie*, p. 107, 506–7; N. Culpeper, *Culpeper's Directory for Midwives: or, A Guide for Women. The Second Part* (London,1676), p. 212; Heister, *A General System of Surgery*, vol. 1, p. 230–1; R. Temple, *Practice of Physic: Wherein is Attempted a Concise Exposition of the Characters, Symptoms, Causes of Diseases, and Method of Cure, with Formulæ* (London, 1792), pp. 400–1. See also de Moulin, *A Short History of Breast Cancer*, p. 5, 43. On attitudes to diet see Pelling, *The Common Lot*, pp. 38–62; K. Albala, *Eating Right in the Renaissance* (Berkeley, Los Angeles, CA and London: University of California Press, 2002); see also R. Porter, 'Spreading Medical Enlightenment. The Popularization of Medicine in Georgian England, and its Paradoxes', in R. Porter (ed.), *The Popularization of Medicine: 1650–1850* (London: Routledge, 1992), p. 215.
7. Pearson, *Practical Observations*, p. 44.
8. Wear, *Knowledge and Practice*, pp. 155–6, 169–78.
9. Guillemeau, *A Worthy Treatise*, p. 43–4; Guillemeau, *A Treatise*, sig. O2v–O3.
10. Ball, *The Female Physician*, p. 88.
11. Gentlemen of the Faculty, *The Medical Museum: or, A Repository of Cases, Experiments, Researches, and Discoveries, Collected at Home and Abroad*, vol. 3 (London, 1764), p. 376; Bayfield, *Enchiridion Medicum*, p. 293. For mild milk diet in avoiding heating of 'the machine', see Wallis, *The Art of Preventing Diseases*, p. 764. On the Arabic tradition, with similar suggestions in English, see M. i. M. Jighmini, *Short Canons of the Art of Physic, Terjuma canoonché Mahmood Cheghmeny der elm tebb. Being a Compendium, Both of Theory and Practice. Written Originally in Arabic* (Calcutta, 1782), pp. 124–5.
12. Ball, *The Female Physician*, p. 88, and nearly identically Gentleman of the Faculty, *Every Lady Her Own Physician*, pp. 69–70. See also Buchan, *Domestic Medicine*, p. 602.
13. Rowley, *Seventy Four Select Cases*, p. 19.
14. H. Manning, *Modern Improvements in the Practice of Surgery* (London, 1780), p. 95. On vegetarianism see D. G. Charlton, *New Images of the Natural in France. A Study in European Cultural History 1750–1800* (Cambridge: Cambridge University Press, 1984), pp.

29–30, 202; Wear, *Knowledge and Practice*, p. 173; R. Porter, *Flesh in the Age of Reason* (London: Penguin, 2003), p 239.

15. Hippocrates, *Hippocrates's Treatise*, p. 40; Hill, *Plain and Useful Directions*, pp. 4–8. While Galenism was discredited, Hippocrates 'survived as a living symbol', Nutton, *Ancient Medicine*, p. 15.

16. Ball, *The Female Physician*, p. 105, and again, found in Gentleman of the Faculty, *Every Lady Her Own Physician*, pp. 74–5. Violent exercise was to be avoided: Manning, *Modern Improvements*, p. 95. See also Buchan, *Domestic Medicine*, p. 602.

17. Galen cured a woman with breast cancer with 'a year's course of purgation'. Nutton, *Ancient Medicine*, p. 35. See also S. Kuriyama, 'The Forgotten Fear of Excrement', *Journal of Medieval and Early Modern Studies*, 38:3 (2008), pp. 413–42.

18. W. Salmon, *Medicina Practica, or, Practical Physick Shewing the Method of Curing the Most Usual Diseases Happening to Humane Bodies* (London, 1692), p. 28; Culpeper, *Culpeper's Directory*, p. 213. This was often repeated before him as well as after. Examples: Wecker, *A Compendious Chyrurgerie*, pp. 107, 506; MacBride, *Methodical Introduction*, pp. 626–7; Jighmini, *Short Canons*, pp. 124–5; D. Porter and Roy Porter, *Patient's Progress. Doctors and Doctoring in Eighteenth-Century England* (Stanford, CA: Stanford University Press, 1989), pp. 160–1, 170–1; Nutton, *Ancient Medicine*, p. 35.

19. On the Helmontian attack on purges, see Wear, *Knowledge and Practice*, pp. 378–84.

20. Wallis, *The Art of Preventing Diseases*, p. 762. Bleeding was often recommended as part of good palliative care. *London Practice of Physic*, p. 181. On the meanings of blood in early modern England in general, see Paster, *The Body Embarrassed*, p. 64–112.

21. Ball, *The Female Physician*, p. 90.

22. Inhabitant of Bath, *John v. 6. Wilt Thou be Made Whole, or, The Virtues and Efficacy of the Water of Glastonbury in the County of Somerset* (London, 1751), pp. 19–21; Wiseman, *Eight Chirurgical Treatises*, pp. 176, 179.

23. K. Olsen, *Daily Life in 18th-Century England* (Westport, CT and London: Greenwood Press, 1999), pp. 276–8; *London Practice of Physic*, p. 182; Guy, *A Select Number of Schirrhus and Cancerous Cases*, p. 1; F. Haslam, *From Hogarth to Rowlandson* (Liverpool: Liverpool University Press, 1996), p. 194.

24. *Medical Observations and Inquiries*, vol. 4, p. 359.

25. In 'Female Disorders', Coates provides a thorough general account of medications for women's illnesses in the eighteenth century, and on pp. 67–91 discusses the medications for breast cancer.

26. N. D. Jewson, 'Medical Knowledge and the Patronage System in the 18th Century England', *Sociology*, 8:3 (1974), pp. 369–85.

27. Coates, 'Female Disorders', p. 58. That the disease was seen as an individual problem and to be treated individually is due to Galen's victory over the so called methodists. Nutton, *Ancient Medicine*, p. 239.

28. N. Grew, *Musaeum Regalis Societatis, or, A Catalogue and Description of the Natural and Artificial Rarities Belonging to the Royal Society* (London, 1685), p. 320.

29. Pliny, *The Historie of the World*, pp. 46, 275–6, 266 [*sic*, pages misnumbered].

30. C. Estienne, *Maison Rustique, or The Countrey Farme, translated into English by Richard Surflet* (London, 1616), pp. 213, 224; J. Gerard, *The Herball or Generall Historie of Plantes. Gathered by Iohn Gerarde of London Master in Chirurgerie, Very Much Enlarged and Amended by Thomas Iohnson Citizen and Apothecarye of London* (London, 1633), chapter 198; W. Bullein, *Bulleins Bulwarke of Defence Against All Sicknesse, Soarenesse, and Woundes That Doe Dayly Assaulte Mankinde* (London, 1579/1652, ff. 30, 40; T.

Lupton, *A Thousand Notable Things, of Sundry Sortes Wherof Some Are Wonderfull, Some Straunge, Some Pleasant, Diuers Necessary, a Great Sort Profitable and Many Very Precious* (London, 1579), p. 98; de Moulin, *A Short History of Breast Cancer*, p. 17.

31. Young, *Minutes*, pp. xiv–xv; Receipt-Book, BL, Sloane MS 1481, f. 8v; K. Digby, *Choice and Experimented Receipts in Physick and Chirurgery, as also Cordial and Distilled Waters and Spirits, Perfumes, and Other Curiosities*, 2nd edn (London, 1675), pp. 36–7; interesting medications also on pp. 62–3, 66–7 and in his K. Digby, *A Choice Collection of Rare Secrets and Experiments in Philosophy as Also Rare and Unheard-of Medicines, Menstruums and Alkahests: With the True Secret of Vol.atilizing the Fixt Salt of Tartar* (London, 1682), pp. 229–30, 231–2, 232–3, 264–5.

32. A. Chute, *Tabacco* (London, 1595), pp. 25–7, 43–4; E. Gardiner, *The Triall of Tabacco Wherein, His Worth is Most Worthily Expressed* (London, 1610), p. 46; G. Everard, *Panacea, or, The Universal Medicine Being a Discovery of the Wonderfull Vertues of Tobacco Taken in a Pipe: With its Operation and Use Both in Physick and Chyrurgery* (London, 1659), p. 43; Barbette, *Thesaurus Chirurgiae*, p. 123.

33. U. von Hutten, *Of the Wood Called Guaiacum That Healeth the Frenche Pockes, and Also Healeth the Goute in the Feete, the Stoone, the Palsey, Lepree, Dropsy, Fallynge Euyll, and Other Dyseases* (London, 1536), f. 66; Wear, *Knowledge & Practice*, p. 71. On national aspects of the debate on medications, see ibid., pp. 72–8. See also H. Green, *Wood, Craft, Culture, History* (New York and London: Viking, 2006), pp. 35–6.

34. R. Fludd, *Mosaicall Philosophy Grounded Upon the Essentiall Truth, or Eternal Sapience / Written First in Latin and Afterwards Thus Rendred Into English by Robert Fludd, Esq* (London, 1659), pp. 291–2. 'Mummy' was ideally made of mummies ground to dust, but was often also 'faked'. On Egyptian mummies made for medication, see W. Lithgow: *The Totall Discourse, of the Rare Adventures, and Painefull Peregrinations of Long Nineteen Yeares Trauayles* (London, 1632), pp. 309–10. Thanks to Eva Johanna Holmberg for pointing out this source to me. Schwyzer discusses the mummy trade and the English response to it in Philip Schwyzer, 'Mummy is Become Merchandise: Literature and the Anglo-Egyptian Mummy Trade in the Seventeenth Century', in G. MacLean (ed.), *Re-Orienting the Renaissance. Cultural Exchanges with the East* (Basingstoke and New York: Palgrave, 2005), pp. 66–87. On medical cannibalism in early modern culture, see especially R. Sugg, *Mummies, Cannibals and Vampires. The History of Corpse Medicine from the Renaissance to the Victorians* (London and New York: Routledge, 2011) and L. Noble, *Medicinal Cannibalism in Early Modern English Literature and Culture* (Basingstoke and New York: Palgrave, 2011); K. Arnold, *Cabinets for the Curious. Looking Back at Early English Museums* (Aldershot and Burlington: Ashgate, 2006), p. 135, 154 note 3, and R. Sugg, 'Good Physic but Bad Food': Early Modern Attitudes to Medicinal Cannibalism and Its Suppliers', *Social History of Medicine*, 19:2 (2006), pp. 225–40; M. A. Katritzky, *Women, Medicine and Theatre, 1500–1750* (Aldershot and Burlington, VT: Ashgate, 2007), p. 132.

35. Nisbet, *An Inquiry*, pp. 205–6; *Medical Commentaries*, vol. 1, p. 12. *Petroleum Barbadense*, Barbados tar, another American import, used externally, and was found more powerful than hemlock – on which more later. *Medical Commentaries*, vol. 6, pp. 372, 375.

36. Buchan, *Domestic Medicine*, p. 605. See also *Modern Family Physician*, pp. 221, 401–2.

37. On carrot poultices, T. Marryat, *The Art of Healing, or a New Practice of Physic*, 5th edn (Birmingham, 1776), p. 326; Cornwell, *The Domestic Physician*, p. 531; Culpeper, *Culpeper's English Physician*, p. 183; Latta, *A Practical System of Surgery*, vol. 1, p. 144; Rowley, *A Treatise on the Management of Female Breasts*, p. 43; *Medical Observations and*

Inquiries, vol. 4, pp. 362, 365–6. Carrot was used as a medication in ancient medicine, Nutton, *Ancient Medicine*, p. 172.

38. I am fully aware of the criticism that concepts such as 'revolution' have received in this and other similar contexts. However, I see the changes which took place in medicine as so great that I have decided – after long resistance – to use the term here. It should not be read as suggesting either a teleological notion of progress or an essentialized understanding of the 'triumph' of early modern medicine, but merely, as it were, as a dramatic change. These changes, revolutions, are always, born in a long process. I believe that the nature of historical change is slow and sporadic. As William Sewell Jr puts it, 'the world may prove quite recalcitrant to our attempts to shape it', in W. H. Sewell, *Logics of History. Social Theory and Social Transformation* (Chicago, IL and London: University of Chicago Press, 2005), p. 191; for more on the nature of change in cultures, pp. 189–96. We could easily follow Bruce Moran, who points out that the Scientific Revolution was 'a subjective reevalution of experiences that had been around for a very long time'. B. T. Moran, *Distilling Knowledge. Alchemy, Chemistry, and the Scientific Revol.ution* (Cambridge, MA, and London: Harvard University Press, 2005), p. 99. See also S. Shapin, *A Social History of Truth: Civility and Science in Seventeenth-Century England* (Chicago, IL: University of Chicago Press, 1994); Shapin, *The Scientific Revolution* (Chicago, IL: University of Chicago Press, 1996).

39. Moran, *Distilling Knowledge*, p. 89. Webster called chemists 'the Chemical Evangelists', in C. Webster, *The Great Instauration. Science, Medicine and Reform 1626–1660* (London: Duckworth, 1975), pp. 273–4. Wear considers Paracelsians and Helmontians as the agents of change in early modern medicine, and indeed they stirred up discussion about cancer as well. Wear, *Knowledge and Practice*, pp. 5, 39. On the Helmontians in general see ibid., pp. 353–433; on their remedies in particular, ibid., pp. 387–98. On magnetism, L. Kassell, 'Magic, Alchemy and the Medical Economy in Early Modern England: The Case of Robert Fludd's Magnetical Medicine' in M. S. R. Jenner and P. Wallis (eds) *Medicine and the Market in England and Its Colonies, c. 1450–c. 1850* (Basingstoke and New York: Palgrave, 2007), p. 107. See also L. Kassell, *Medicine and Magic in Elizabethan London. Simon Forman: Astrologer, Alchemist, and Physician* (Oxford: Clarendon Press, 2005), esp. pp. 6–9; Moran, *Distilling Knowledge*, esp. 72–9.

40. H. M. Herwig, *The Art of Curing Sympathetically, or Magnetically*, orig. in Latin (London, 1700); pp. 16–17. Wear, *Knowledge and Practice*, pp. 360–1. For an excellent introduction to Paracelsus's understanding of the origin of illness, see Moran, *Distilling Knowledge*, pp. 74–7. On p. 85 he comments on the sixteenth-century projects of several authors to link Paracelsian ideas with old traditions; he discusses Helmont (as a vitalist) on pp. 89–94.

41. Webster, *The Great Instauration*, pp. 273–4.

42. R. Johnson, *Praxis Medicinae Reformata: = or, The Practice of Physick Reformed Being an Epitome of the Whole Art* (London, 1700), p. iv; M. Cavendish, *Ground of Natural Philosophy Divided Into Thirteen Parts* (London, 1668), p. 144. On cancer as 'illness of resolution', see W. Russell, *A Physical Treatise Grounded, not Upon Tradition, Nor Phancy, but Experience* (London, 1684), p. 68.

43. See for example J. Headrich, *Arcana Philosophia, or, Chymical Secrets Containing the Noted and Useful Chymical Medicines* (London, 1697), pp. 24, 25, 49. Wear posits that it was more difficult for the layman to understand chemical medicine than Galenic medicine. A. Wear, 'The Popularization of Medicine in Early Modern England', in R. Porter (ed.), *The Popularization of Medicine 1650–1850* (London and New York: Routledge,

1992), p. 20. See also R. O'Day, *The Professions in Early Modern England, 1450–1800: Servants of the Commonweal* (Harlow etc.: Longman, 2000), p. 226.

44. Chemists of course used plants as well. For example, Thomason recommended lunaria in G. Thomson, *Ortho-Methodoz Itro-Chymike: Or the Direct Method of Curing Chymically Wherein is Conteined [sic] the Original Matter, and Principal Agent of All Natural Bodies* (London, 1675), p. 143. Below I discuss the use of hemlock, the special cancer medicine of the Helmontians. Moran, *Distilling Knowledge*, pp. 77–8.

45. Paracelsus, *A Hundred and Fouretene Experiments and Cures of the Famous Physitian Philippus Aureolus Theophrastus Paracelsus* (London, 1596), p. 4.

46. Moran, *Distilling Knowledge*, p. 93.

47. Culpeper, *Culpeper's Directory*, p. 213. This repeated Bright's advice: T. Bright, *A Treatise, Wherein is Declared the Sufficiencie of English Medicines, for Cure of All Diseases, Cured with Medicines* (London, 1615), p. 46. This recipe survived for a long time, as it was reprinted for example in Culpeper, *The English Physician*, p. 159.

48. Galenists and nightshade, see: Barrough, *The Methode of Phisicke*, pp. 276, 277. Moulin, *A Short History of Breast Cancer*, p. 50, mentions the Hungerford case. Wiseman advised using the oil of frogs cooked with butter in their mouths. He also recommended frogspawn water in summer. Wiseman, *Eight Chirurgical Treatises*, p. 171. Nightshade was also used in France: C. Deshaies-Gendron, *Enquiries into the Nature, Knowledge, and Cure of Cancers ... done out of French* (London, 1701), p. 118–9, mentions that it was used by his uncle, the Abbot Gendron. Thomas Gataker used Nightshade, both Garden Nightshade and Deadly Nightshade, on several patients, but found it of no use; for nine case histories, see T. Gataker, *Essays on Medical Subjects, Originally Printed Separately; to which is now Prefixed an Introduction relating to the Use of Hemlock and Corrosive Sublimate; and to the Application of Caustic Medicines in Cancerous Disorders* (London, 1764), pp. 54–69.

49. Empiricism was a long-lasting process in the history of Western natural history and science in general. As Bruce Moran posits, alchemical knowledge was an important part of the heritage which early modern science incorporated into itself. De Moran, *Distilling Knowledge*. Early modern science saw no need to completely renounce the occult, and the 'old' types of science and new empiricism continued to coexist. There were feverish proponents of the new kind of science in all fields of natural history, for instance, and as for example David Freedberg has demonstrated, botany was a field where Galilean theories and an emphasis on experimentation rapidly gained a footing. D. Freedberg, *The Eye of the Lynx. Galileo, His Friends, and the Beginnings of Modern Natural History* (Chicago, IL and London: University of Chicago Press, 2002), passim, esp. 3.

50. Wear finds little change in medicine 'from the mid-sixteenth to the mid-seventeenth century': Wear, *Knowledge and Practice*, p. 5. Later he points out that '[a]lthough therapeutics has undergone vast changes since the time of the ancient Greeks, preventive medicine has changed much less. Many of the topics around which the advice has been organized, such as food, exercise and emotional well-being, have remained the same, as have some of the assumptions behind the advice. They include the existence of a relationship between people and the food they eat and the environment they live in, and the need for both food and environment to be clean, uncorrupted and 'natural'. Ibid., pp. 155–6.

51. O'Day, *The Professions*, p. 225.

52. Such a suggestion could be made if one believed blood was the origin of cancer. J. Glanvill, *Plus Ultra, or, The Progress and Advancement of Knowledge since the Days of Aristotle* (London, 1668), pp. 17–8; J. Glanvill, *Essays on Several Important Subjects in Philosophy and Religion* (London, 1676), p. 6. Henry Stubbe, a Galenist, cited and criticized Glan-

vill for misunderstanding and actually confusing the techniques of blood transfusions and injections. H. Stubbe, *Legends No Histories, or, A Specimen of Some Animadversions upon The History of the Royal Society* (London, 1670), pp. 116–7.

53. Coates, 'Female Disorders', pp. 58–9.
54. De Moulin, *A Short History of Breast Cancer*, p. 43. On the use of electricity, Porter and Porter, *Patient's Progress*, p. 171.
55. J. Leake, *Medical Instructions towards the Prevention and Cure of Chronic Diseases Peculiar to Women*, 5th edn, vol. 1 (London, 1781), pp. 357–8; A. Duncan, *Medical Cases, Selected from the Records of the Public Dispensary at Edinburgh: with Remarks and Observations; being the Substance of Case-Lectures, Delivered during the Years 1776–7*, 2nd edn (Edinburgh, 1781), pp. 106–7, 111–4. White considered the results of the tests on electricity to be promising. White, *Practical Surgery*, pp. 45–6.
56. Leake, *Medical Instructions*, p. 350.
57. A. Duncan, *Lectures on the Theory and Practice of Medicine*, 3rd edn (Edinburgh, 1781), p. 202.
58. Duncan, *Medical Cases*, pp. 106–7, 111–4; White, *Practical Surgery*, pp. 45–6.
59. Duncan, *Medical Cases*, pp. 111–4. The same patient was also given hemlock.
60. Interestingly, Pearson considered it indifferent whether one operated a large or a small cancer. Much more important than the age of the tumour was to remove all cancerous parts. Pearson, *Practical Observations*, p. 52.
61. Ewart, *The History of Two Cases*, p. v. Townsend was convinced of Ewart's findings, having witnessed a treatment in Bath. Townsend, *A Guide to Health*, pp. 464–5.
62. Ewart, *The History of Two Cases*, pp. 11–12.
63. Ibid., pp. 18–19.
64. Ibid., pp. 19-21, 23, 24, 25–7.
65. T. Philipot, *Self-Homicide-Murther, or, Some Antidotes and Arguments Gleaned Out of the Treasuries of Our Modern Casuists and Divines Against that Horrid and Reigning Sin of Self-Murther* (London, 1674), pp. 16–17. In M. Cavendish, *Observations upon Experimental Philosophy to Which is Added the Description of a New Blazing World* (London, 1666), pp. 82–3 the Duchess of Newcastle, noted her scepticism about the possibilities of the new science in promising a cure for all diseases. In fact she believed there could be no such thing as universal medicine. She admitted that there might be ways to cure diseases such as cancers and the like, but was pessimistic about the possibility of curing illnesses caused by 'the decay of the vital parts'.
66. Burrows, *A New Practical Essay on Cancers*, pp. 58–60.
67. Marryat, *All the Prescriptions*, pp. 135–6; Marryat, *The Art of Healing*, pp. 325–6; White, *Practical Surgery*, p. 44.
68. Buchan, *Domestic Medicine*, pp. 602–3. Similar suggestion: G. A. Gordon, *The Complete English Physician; or, An Universal Library of Family Medicines* (London, 1779), p. 19.
69. J. Higgs, *A Practical Essay on the Cure of Venereal, Scorbutic, Arthritic, Leprous, Scrophulous, and Cancerous Disorders* (London, 1755), pp. 31–2.
70. Störck's book included seven cases of breast illnesses, most of which were diagnosed as schirrhi. All these patients were cured. Two of the patients were diagnosed with cancer, both of whom died. Störck attested, however, that hemlock was useful even in true cancer, since it improved the condition of the patients, and removed the smell of ulcers. A. von Störck, *An Essay on Hemlock. Wherein, from a Variety of Sases, the Efficacy of this Plant, in the Cure of Cancers ... is Fully Demonstrated. Newly Translated from the Latin, by F. H. Physician* (Aberdeen, 1762), pp. 59–60. His breast cases: pp. 12–17 (case II, schir-

rhus, cured), pp. 18–19 (case III, real schirrhus, cured), pp. 19–21 (case IV, ulcerated schirrhus, cured), pp. 26–7 (case VII, lump from accident, cured), pp. 27–33 (case VIII, latent cancer later ulcerated, died), pp. 37–40 (case XI, cancer, died), pp. 46–7 (case XIV, schirrhus, apparently cured). See also Manning, *Modern Improvements*, pp. 95–6.

71. Störck, *An Essay on Hemlock*, pp. 4, 6–7. Experimenting on animals was common, and followed ancient example, Nutton, *Ancient Medicine*, p. 231.

72. Astruc, *A Treatise on the Diseases of Women*, vol. 3, p. 357; Tissot, *Advice to People in General*, p. 225, footnote; *Compendium of Physic*, pp. 247–8, only recommended hemlock as a palliative medicine. Frewen suggested that hemlock's failure to produce similarly wonderful effects in England as in Germany might be due to the different climate in which the plant grew. Frewen, *Physiologia*, pp. 433–6. In a similar vein, Townsend considered hemlock an excellent remedy in Germany and Spain, but noted that in England, where hemlock was of different quality, a more useful plant was 'the flores martiales' (*ferrum ammoniacae*). Townsend, *A Guide to Health*, pp. 463–4.

73. Guy, *Practical Observations*, pp. 41–51. Similar: J. Hill, *Cases in Surgery, Particularly, of Cancers, and Disorders of the Head from External Violence* (Edinburgh, 1772), p. 29; Marryat, *All the Prescriptions*, p. 135; Marryat, *The Art of Healing*, p. 326; Burrows, *A New Practical Essay on Cancers*, pp. 65–70; Aitken, *Principles of Midwifery*, p. 65.

74. Dominiceti, *Medical Anecdotes*, pp. 372–4 (footnote).

75. Ibid., p. 374.

76. *London Practice of Physic*, p. 185. Others: Manning, *Modern Improvements*, pp. 95–6; Ball, *The Female Physician*, pp. 98–101; Gentleman of the Faculty, *Every Lady her own Physician*, pp. 72–4; Buchan, *Domestic Medicine*, p. 605; MacBride, *Methodical Introduction*, p. 626; Duncan, *Medical Cases*, p. 113. See also *Modern Family Physician*, pp. 220–1; Bissett, Cases, Wellcome MS 1964, f. 437; Gentlemen of the Faculty, *The Medical Museum*, vol. 3, pp. 566–7, 569; Nicolson in *Medical Observations and Inquiries*, vol. 4, pp. 359–62, 366; Morley, *The Eighteenth Edn*, pp. 34.

77. J. O. Justamond, *An Account of the Methods Pursued in the Treatment of Cancerous and Schirrhous Disorders, and other Indurations* (London, 1780), pp. 29–30.

78. Gentlemen of the Faculty, *The Medical Museum*, vol. 2, pp. 204–5.

79. Duden, *The Woman Beneath the Skin*, pp. 87–8.

80. Pelling, *The Common Lot*, p. 29; E. Cohen, 'The Expression of Pain in the Later Middle Ages: Deliverance, Acceptance and Infamy', in F. Egmond and R. Zwijnenberg (eds), *Bodily Extremities. Preoccupations with the Human Body in Early Modern European Culture* (Aldershot and Burlington, VT: Ashgate, 2003), pp. 195–219; E. Cohen, *The Modulated Scream. Pain in Late Medieval Culture* (Chicago, IL and London: University of Chicago Press, 2010). See also Porter and Porter, *Patient's Progress*, pp. 163–5; K. Johannisson, *Kroppens tunna tkal. Sex essäer om kropp, historia och dultur* (Stockholm: Nordstedts, 1997), pp. 69–73, 79; E. F. Crane, '"I Have Suffer'd Much Today": The Defining Force of Pain in Early America', in R. Hoffman, M. Sobel and F. J. Teute (eds), *Through a Glass Darkly. Reflections on Personal Identity in Early America* (Chapel Hill, CT and London: Omohundro Institute of Early American History & Culture and the University of North Carolina Press, 1997), pp. 370–403. Examples include: A. Searle (ed.), *Barrington Family Letters 1628–1632*, Camden Fourth Series, 28 (London: Royal Historical Society, 1983), p. 200; M. H. Nicolson (ed.), S. Hutton (rev. ed.), *The Conway Letters. The Correspondence of Anne, Viscountess Conway, Henry More, and their Friends 1642–1684* (Oxford: Clarendon Press, 1992). On Anne Conway, see also Porter and Porter, *In Sickness and In Health*, pp. 124–7; M. Nurminen, 'Anatomiaa ja ihmetekoja.

Thomas Willis, Valentine Greatrakes ja parantamisen monet muodot restauraatioajan Englannissa' (PhD Dissertation, University of Helsinki, 2012); Letters from Mrs. Carter to Mrs Vesey, Letter 4, Deal, Dec. 6, 1763, in E. Carter and C. Talbot (1809): *A Series of Letters between Mrs. Elizabeth Carter and Miss Catherine Talbot, from the year 1742 to 1770. To which are Added, Letters from Mrs. Elizabeth Carter to Mrs. Vesey, between the Years 1763 and 1787*, vol. 1. (London, 1809), pp. 230–2. On medieval religious meanings of pain and suffering, see C. W. Bynum, *Holy Feast and Holy Fast. The Religious Significance of Food to Medieval Women* (Berkeley, CA: University of California Press, 1987), pp. 209–10; C. W. Bynum, *Fragmentation and Redemption. Essays on Gender and the Human Body in Medieval Religion* (New York: Zone Books, 1992), pp. 131, 182. On the history of sedation and related issues, see R. Rey, *The History of Pain* (Cambridge, MA and London: Harvard University Press, 1993/8), pp. 64–6, 82–5, 125–31. See also Porter and Porter, *In Sickness and In Health*, p. 102; Pelling, *The Common Lot*, pp. 222–4; O'Day, *The Professions*, p. 217; On pain and surgery, Wear, *Knowledge and Practice*, pp. 247–8.

81. Mustow, Commonplace book, BL Sloane MS 2117, ff. 83v, 110.
82. J. Banister, *An Antidotarie Chyrurgicall Containing Great Varietie and Choice of All Sorts of Medicines That Commonly Fall Into the Chyrurgions Use*, pp. 41, 165.
83. Cornwell, *The Domestic Physician*, p. 531.
84. According to Sykes and Bunker, Henry Hill Hickman was the first to attempt surgical anaesthesia (with carbon dioxide) in 1820s. K. Sykes and J. Bunker, *Anaesthesia and the Practice of Medicine: Historical Perspectives* (London: Royal Society of Medicine Press, 2007), p. 8. Ether was first used in an operation in October 1846. J. S. Olson, *Bathsheba's Breast. Women, Cancer & History* (Baltimore, MD and London: Johns Hopkins University Press, 2002), pp. 54–5. See also D. B. Morris, *The Culture of Pain* (Berkeley, Los Angeles, CA and London: California University Press, 1991/3), pp. 61, 64.
85. Latta, *A Practical System of Surgery*, vol. 2, pp. 533–4.
86. Mustow, Commonplace book, BL Sloane MS 2117, f. 83v.
87. Laudanum was seen as so dangerous that it was strictly denied to children under two years of age. For them, diacodium was considered the safe option. See Bath & Co., *A Description of the Names and Qualities of those Medicinal Compositions Contained in the Domestic Medicine Chests; with an Account of their Several Uses, and the Quantities Proper to Give at Each Dose* (London, [c. 1775]), p. 20. Wear, *Knowledge & Practice*, p. 246.
88. Rey, *The History of Pain*, pp. 92–3.
89. Mustow, Commonplace book, BL, Sloane MS 2117, f. 101.
90. Hill, *Cases in Surgery*, pp. 23–4.
91. The use of opiates had continued from antiquity; it was known for example to New Kingdom Egyptians and ancient Greeks. King, *Hippocrates' Woman*, pp. 118–20.
92. Mustow, Commonplace book, BL, Sloane MS 2117, ff. 83v, 110. On Sydenham's Laudanum, see Rey, *The History of Pain*, pp. 82–5. Porter notes that there were many substances such as 'tea, coffee, tobacco, sugar … bitters, tonics, narcotics, sedatives, quack, patent and proprietary medicines' which were considered poisonous. Porter, *Flesh in the Age of Reason*, p. 403.
93. R. Porter, *English Society in the 18th Century*, rev. edn (London: Penguin, 1991), p. 16. Also in Porter and Porter, *In Sickness and in Health*, p. 102. Porter suggests the eighteenth century as a century of dependency. On dependency and addiction in the eighteenth century, see Porter, *Flesh in the Age of Reason*, pp. 374–97. For the first time, Europeans were becoming addicted on a larger scale, and especially alcohol and opiates

were seen as dangerous. The early eighteenth century has often been called the Gin Age, so strong was the influence of the new distilled drink. P. Earle, *A City Full of People. Men and Women of London 1650–1750* (London: Methuen, 1994), p. 6.

94. Porter provocatively observes 'that the "age of feeling" was arguably lowering the pain threshold'. Porter, *Flesh in the Age of Reason*, p. 403.

95. Rey, *The History of Pain*, pp. 125–7.

96. J. Jones, *The Mysteries of Opium Reveal'd* (London, 1700), p. 17. See also Wiseman, *Eight Chirurgical Treatises*, pp. 171.

97. Jones, *The Mysteries of Opium*, pp. 19, 322–3, 370.

98. Fearon, *A Treatise on Cancers*, pp. 128–9.

99. G. Young, *A Treatise on Opium, Founded upon Practical Observations* (London, 1753), p. 87. Jones praised opium in Jones, *The Mysteries of Opium*, p. 20. See also Bell, *A System of Surgery*, vol. 1, p. 147.

100. He came to doubt opium's virtues however, when he saw that those who used it died earlier than those who did not use it. Young, *A Treatise on Opium*, pp. 125–6.

101. Cited in Epstein, 'Writing the Unspeakable', pp. 147–8.

102. Hunter, *The Case Books*, p. 58.

103. Buchan, *Domestic Medicine*, p. 606. Identical advice in Cornwell, *The Domestic Physician*, p. 535; Mansey, *The Practical Physician*, p. 379, likewise characterizes opium as 'a kind of solace'. See also Fearon, *A Treatise on Cancers*, pp. 74–5; Manning, *Modern Improvements*, p. 97; Latta, *A Practical System of Surgery*, p. 148–9, 154; Heister, *A General System of Surgery*, vol. 1, pp. 231. Le Clerc, *The Compleat Surgeon*, p. 166.

104. Fearon, *A Treatise on Cancers*, p. xv.

105. Pearson, *Principles of Surgery*, pp. 246–7.

106. Wear, *Knowledge and Practice*, pp. 248–50; O'Day, *The Professions*, p. 226, provides a slightly less optimistic view. A great role in the dissemination of information was played of course above all by publishing, but also by institutions such as the Royal Society. Webster, *The Great Instauration*, pp. 88–99.

107. Beckett, *New Discoveries*, p. 54.

108. Heister, *A General System of Surgery*, vol. 1, pp. 228–9.

109. Rowley, *Practical Treatise*, pp. 53–4.

110. Rowley, *Seventy Four Select Cases*, pp. 15–16.

111. It is no wonder not everyone liked what he had to say. There was a fierce attack against his 'pulvis mineralis' and his method of verifying his cases. He wrote an equally severe response to this criticism, and published it as W. Rowley, *An answer to the criticism in the Monthly review for October 1779, on a pamphlet lately published, called Seventy-four cases* (London, 1779), pp. 3–4. He was then in turn fiercely attacked by his enemies.

112. Sixteenth century: Guillemeau, *A Worthy Treatise*, p. 1587; Wecker, *A compendious Chyrurgerie*, p. 506. Seventeenth century: Barbette, *Thesaurus Chirurgiae*, p. 124; Beckett, *New Discoveries*, pp. 53–4. See also Aitken, *Principles of Midwifery*, p. 65; Burrows, *A New Practical Essay on Cancers*, pp. 58–71; Thornton, *The Philosophy of Medicine*, vol. 5, pp. 414–5. See also de Moulin, *A Short History of Breast Cancer*, pp. 14–15, 24.

113. Justamond, *An Account*, pp. 18, 33, 35. In France, Monsieur Le Febure had noted that the only remedy for cancer was indeed arsenic. It was taken inwardly, and could be used outwardly as a wash. See Society in Edinburgh, *Medical and Philosophical Commentaries ... vol. 4* (London, 1776), pp. 55, 59, 60.

114. Rowley, *Seventy Four Select Cases*, pp. 18–9.

115. Rowley, *A Treatise on the Management of Female Breasts*, p. 32.

116. For example Dionis, *A Course of Chirurgical Operations*, pp. 253–6 explains the different techniques used in these two operations.

117. Norford, *An Essay*, pp. 114, 118.

118. Payne, *With Words and Knives*, pp. 103–23.

119. Dionis, *A Course of Chirurgical Operations*, p. 243.

120. Guillemeau, *A Worthy Treatise*, p. 49; Nutton, *Ancient Medicine*, pp. 23, 35.

121. Wecker, *A Compendious Chyrurgerie*, p. 107. Barrough, *The Methode of Phisicke*, p. 274; Banister, *The Workes*, p. 59. Guillemeau, *A Worthy Treatise*, p. 62. Bayfield, *Enchiridion Medicum*, p. 293. See also P. E. Pormann and E. Savage-Smith, *Medieval Islamic Medicine* (Washington, DC: Georgetown University Press, 2007), pp. 107, 130.

122. Beier, *Sufferers & Healers*, pp. 82, 84.

123. Anon., *The Compleat Doctoress: or, A Choice Treatise of All Diseases Insident to Women … Faithfully Translated Out of Latine into English for a Common Good* (London, 1656), p.50. See also Deshaies-Gendron, *Enquiries*, pp. 82, 102; Maynwaringe, *The Frequent, but Unsuspected Progress of Pains*, pp. 195–6; Culpeper, *Culpeper's Directory*, p. 212. See also Culpeper, *The English Physician*, pp. 158–9. On Culpeper and his political programme, which included ideologically raising the male body above the female one, see Fissell, *Vernacular Bodies*, pp. 4, 135–56. Wear notes that he was probably a Leveller; he wanted the poor to have access to chief local medications. Wear, 'The Popularization of Medicine', p. 31. On Hippocratic tradition and breast cancer, see de Moulin, *A Short History of Breast Cancer*, p. 2.

124. B. Saviard, *Observations in Surgery: Being a Collection of One Hundred and Twenty Eight Different Cases … Written Originally in French … translation … by J. S. Surgeon* (London, 1740), pp. 124–5.

125. Barbette, *Thesaurus Chirurgiae*, p. 124.

126. Moyle, *The Experienced Chirurgion*, pp. 48–9.

127. Rowley, *Practical Treatise*, p. iv. Medications such as 'Pieces of veal, pullets, toads, hemlock, night-shade &c' cured no-one and merely hastened death. Ibid., p. vii. See also Rowley, *A Treatise on the Management of Female Breasts*, pp. 6, 9–10. More on his pessimism relating the possibility of a cure, Ibid., pp. 12–13.

128. D. Ingram, *Practical Cases and Observations in Surgery, with Remarks Highly Proper, not only for the Improvement of All Young Surgeons, but Also for the Direction of Such as are Farther Advanced* (London, 1751), p. xi.

129. Dionis, *A Course of Chirurgical Operations*, p. 250.

130. Brookes, *The General Practice of Physic*, p. 122; van Swieten, *An Abridgement*, p. 428; Latta, *A Practical System of Surgery*, vol. 1, p. 154. In volume 2, he added, however, that if the tumour was loose and not connected, it should be operated on. Ibid., vol. 2, p. 512; Garengeot, *A Treatise of Chirurgical Operations*, p. 292; Le Dran, *The Operations in Surgery*, pp. 298, 300; Aitken, *Principles of Midwifery*, p. 65. See also the second edn of the work, 1785, pp. 122, 124; Wallis, *The Art of Preventing Diseases*, p. 762; Pearson, *Practical Observations*, p. 44; Cornwell, *The Domestic Physician*, pp. 527–8. Duncan, *Medical Cases*, p. 109.

131. Boulton, *A System of Rational and Practical Chirurgery*, p. 114; *London Practice of Physic*, p. 184.

132. Duncan, *Medical Cases*, p. 110. Pearson considered this to be corrosive; it did not always cause cancer, but provided the means of spreading the disease. Pearson, *Principles of Surgery*, pp. 236–7.

133. Duncan, *Medical Cases*, p. 111.

134. Bell, *A System of Surgery*, vol. 5, pp. 170–4.

135. Brookes, *The General Practice of Physic*, p. 122.

136. Buchan, *Domestic Medicine*, p. 603.

137. Ibid.

138. *The Edinburgh Practice*, p. 683.

139. Gooch, *The Chirurgical Works*, vol. 3, pp. 183–4, 187. In B. Gooch, *A Practical Treatise on Wounds and Other Chirurgical Subjects*, vol. 1 (Norwich, 1767), p. 135, he presents the case of a 'noble lady' who had a mastectomy even though affected in such manner, and who had remained well ever since, for more than six years; on pp. 136–7 a case of 'a gentlewoman' who similarly had recovered from a fatal-seeming state.

140. S. Sharp, *A Treatise on the Operations of Surgery, with a Description and Representation of the Instruments Used in Performing Them*, 2nd edn (London, 1739), pp. 130–1.

141. Fearon, *A Treatise on Cancers*, pp. 81–2. Amongst his cases is the one of Elizabeth Auger whom I discuss in more detail later: he deemed her case beyond help, and yet operated – in fact twice. Ibid., pp. 152–5.

142. White, *Practical Surgery*, pp. 367–8.

143. Fearon, *A Treatise on Cancers*, pp. 5–6. Robert White followed Fearon's teachings; he stressed that even if the patient and her friends, when the tumour or tumours were in an indolent stage and painless, thought that an operation might not be necessary because that stage could last for years, it was nevertheless advisable to operate as early as possible because only this could promise 'lasting success'. White, *Practical Surgery*, p. 367.

144. Fearon, *A Treatise on Cancers*, p. 11. Thanks to Raija Vainio for pointing out to me the origin of this quotation in Vergil's *Aeneid* 1, 630.

145. These were the cases of Elizabeth Turner (case III, whom I discuss in the next chapter), and an anonymous pregnant woman (case IV), pp. 141–4.

146. Nisbet, *An Inquiry*, pp. 227–9.

147. Ibid., pp. 230.

148. Nisbet, *An Inquiry*, pp. 232, 258.

149. Pearson, *Principles of Surgery*, pp. 233–4.

150. Nisbet, *The Clinical Guide*, pp. 116.

151. Ibid., pp. 116–7.

152. De Moulin, *A Short History of Breast Cancer*, p. 48; Coates, 'Female Disorders', p. 62.

153. G. Coltman, *An Address to the Public on the Efficacy of Certain Medicines in the Cure of the Venereal Diseases, Scirrhus and Cancer and Ulcerated Legs* (London, 1786), pp. 21–2.

154. Astruc, *A Treatise on the Diseases of Women*, vol. 3, pp. 355–6. Similar pessimism was expressed by Brookes, *The General Practice of Physic*, p. 122.

155. Ball, *The Female Physician*, p. 87.

156. Burrows, *A New Practical Essay on Cancers*, pp. 57–8.

157. Ibid., pp. 71–2.

158. Gooch, *The Chirurgical Works*, vol. 3, p. 186. See also Manning, *Modern Improvements*, p. 90.

159. Wiseman, *Eight Chirurgical Treatises*, p. 172.

160. Gooch, *The Chirurgical Works*, vol. 3, p. 185.

161. Guillemeau, *A Worthy Treatise*, p. 63.

162. Dionis, *A Course of Chirurgical Operations*, p. 253, for example discussed the history of the field. See also de Moulin, *A Short History of Breast Cancer*, p. 23; Yalom, *History of the Breast*, p. 217.

163. Barbette, *Thesaurus Chirurgiae*, p. 124.

164. Van Swieten, *An Abridgement*, p. 444; Heister, *A General System of Surgery*, vol. 2, p. 14, images: table VI, figs 5, 6, hook: table VIII. figs 2, 3.

165. W. Beckett, *Practical Surgery Illustrated and Improved: Being Chirurgical Observations, with Remarks, upon the Most Extraordinary Cases, Cures, and Dissections, made at St. Thomas's Hospital, Southwark* (London, 1740), pp. 161–2. A similar technique was recommended by Dunn, who speaks of a handle being made with the thread, in E. Dunn, *A Compendious and New Method of Performing Chirurgical Operations, Fit for Young Surgeons* (London, 1724), p. 91; and by Brookes, *The General Practice of Physic*, p. 123. Pierre Dionis suggested a single thread would suffice; it was strong enough to sustain the breast and this would 'spare the Patient the Pain'. Dionis, *A Course of Chirurgical Operations*, p. 255. See also J. Handley, *Colloquia Chirurgica: or, The Art of Surgery Epitomiz'd and Made Easy, According to Modern Practice*, 4th edn (London, 1733), p. 70.

166. Beckett, *Practical Surgery*, p. 164.

167. Wiseman, *Eight Chirurgical Treatises*, p. 173. He used the ligature in a case of amputation. Ibid., pp. 180–1.

168. Boulton, *A System of Rational and Practical Chirurgery*, p. 115.

169. Dionis, *A Course of Chirurgical Operations*, p. 255. See also Heister, *A General System of Surgery*, vol. 2, p. 14, and again p. 15.

170. La Vauguion, *A Compleat Body of Chirurgical Operations*, p. 89.

171. De Moulin, *A Short History of Breast Cancer*, p. 46.

172. La Vauguion, *A Compleat Body of Chirurgical Operations*, p. 89; Le Dran, *The Operations in Surgery*, pp. 301–2; Warner, *Cases in Surgery*, p. 356; Fearon, *A Treatise on Cancers*, p. 121; Latta, *A Practical System of Surgery*, vol. 2, p. 512–3; Nisbet, *An Inquiry*, pp. 234–7; Nisbet, *The Clinical Guide*, pp. 259–61; Bell, *A System of Surgery*, vol. 5, pp. 177–80; *The Edinburgh Practice*, p. 683.

173. Bell, *A System of Surgery*, vol. 5, p. 184.

174. Ibid., p. 175.

175. Ibid., p. 189.

176. Sharp, *A Treatise on the Operations of Surgery*, p. 130. Le Dran, *The Operations in Surgery*, tab. X, pp. 453–4.

177. Bell, *A System of Surgery*, vol. 5, pp. 182–3. He noted that ligatures caused hardly any pain but it seems to have been generally considered painful to suture the patient. Ibid., p. 190; Warner, *Cases in Surgery*, pp. 358, 398; Sharp, *A Treatise on the Operations of Surgery*, p. 131.

178. De Moulin, *A Short History of Breast Cancer*, p. 29.

179. Ibid., pp. 30, 45–6.

180. Fearon, *A Treatise on Cancers*, pp. x–xi.

181. Ibid., pp. xi–xii. He was advertised as the inventor of the technique by White, who largely followed Fearon's ideas. White, *Practical Surgery*, p. 370.

182. Fearon, *A Treatise on Cancers*, p. 120.

183. Ibid., pp. 9, 123–5. Fearon mentioned that an identical closing of the wound was to be carried out in castration.

184. Hunter, *The Case Books*, p. 513.

185. Pearson, *Principles of Surgery*, pp. 249–50.

186. White, *Practical Surgery*, p. 368.

187. Bell, *A System of Surgery*, vol. 5, pp. 175–7, 184–5. Similar ideas: Latta, *A Practical System of Surgery*, vol. 2, p. 512.

188. Halsted's radical mastectomy was usually indeed seen as new and 'radical': R. Porter, *Blood and Guts: A Short History of Medicine* (London: Penguin, 2002), p. 126.

189. Bell, *A System of Surgery*, vol. 5, pp. 187–8.

190. Beckett, *New Discoveries*, pp. 46–7.

191. Gooch, *A Practical Treatise on Wounds*, p. 135. Not all were eager to see this as progress. Le Dran was rather pessimistic about the chances of a patient whose cancer had spread to the pectoral muscle. He reminded his readers that even though the pectoral muscle was partly operated upon, he had never seen a cancer spread to the muscle cured. Such a cancer always returned, and killed the patient within a year's time. Le Dran, *The Operations in Surgery*, pp. 304, 305.

192. B. Wilmer, *Cases and Remarks in Surgery* (London, 1779), pp. 119, 124–5.

193. Pearson, *Principles of Surgery*, pp. 250–1.

194. Peyrilhe, *Dissertation on Cancerous Diseases*, p. 107; de Moulin, *A Short History of Breast Cancer*, p. 45; *The Edinburgh Practice*, p. 684.

195. Fearon, *A Treatise on Cancers*, pp. 163, 181.

196. L. Heister, *Medical, Chirurgical, and Anatomical Cases and Observations, transl. from the German original by George Wirgman* (London, 1755), p. 601.

197. De Moulin, *A Short History of Breast Cancer*, p. 29.

3 Women's Agency and Role in Choice of Treatment

1. R. Sweet, 'Women and Civic Life in Eighteenth-Century England', in R. Sweet and P. Lane (eds), *Women and Urban Life in Eighteenth-Century England* (Aldershot and Burlington, VT: Ashgate, 2003), pp. 21–41; D. Simonton, 'Threading the Needle, Pulling the Press: Gender, Skill and the Tools of the Trade in Eighteenth-Century European Towns', *Cultural History*, 1:2 (2012), pp. 180–204.

2. H. Berry, *Gender, Society and Print Culture in Late-Stuart England* (Aldershot and Burlington, VT: Ashgate, 2003), p. 2.

3. On the male gaze, see Robert MacGrath's fascinating *Seeing Her Sex*.

4. Porter and Porter, *Patient's Progress*, pp. 6–7; Wear, 'The Popularization of Medicine', pp. 17, 19. See also Porter and Porter, *Patient's Progress*; Fissell, *Patients, Power, and the Poor*, pp. 16–73; Pelling, *The Common Lot*, pp. 58–9, 242–3; I. Mortimer, 'The Rural Medical Marketplace in Southern England c. 1570–1720' in M. S. R. Jenner and P. Wallis (eds), *Medicine and the Market in England and Its Colonies, c. 1450–c. 1850* (Basingstoke and New York: Palgrave, 2007), pp. 69–87; E. Leong and S. Pennell, 'Recipe Collections and the Currency of Medical Knowledge in the Early Modern 'Medical Marketplace', in ibid., pp. 133–152; Stolberg, *Experiencing Illness*, pp. 58–64; M. Kaartinen, 'Women patients in the medical marketplace in the long eighteenth century England', in A. Montenach and D. Simonton (eds), *Gender and Urban Development. Female Agency in the Eighteenth Century Urban Economy* (London and New York: Routledge 2013, forthcoming).

5. Porter and Porter, *The Patient's Progress*, p. 26–29; Beier, *Sufferers & Healers*, p. 259; N. D. Jewson, 'The Disappearance of the Sick-Man from Medical Cosmology, 1770–1870', *Sociology* 10:2 (1976), pp. 225–244; M. E. Fissell, *Patients, Power, and the Poor in Eighteenth-Century Bristol* (Cambridge: Cambridge University Press, 1991), pp. 148–170; M. E. Fissell, 'Readers, Texts, and Contexts. Vernacular Medical Works in Early Modern England', in R. Porter (ed.) *The Popularization of Medicine 1650–1850* (London and New York: Routledge, 1992, pp. 72–96; D. Armstrong, '*Bodies of Knowledge/Knowledge of Bodies*', in C. Jones and R. Porter (eds) *Reassessing Foucault: Power, Medicine and the*

Body (Abingdon and New York: Routledge, 1994/2006), pp. 17–27; M. Foucault, *The Birth of the Clinic. An Archaeology of Medical Perception*, transl. A. M. Sheridan (London and New York: Routledge, 1973/2006), pp. 15–7, 206–7.

6. K. King, *Jane Barker, Exile. A Literary Career 1676–1725* (Oxford: Oxford University Press, 2000), pp. 103–108 carefully analyses the present and its political meanings. I follow here King's dating of the letter. The letter from I. Barker is included in the Nithsdale collection of letters, misdated for 1739, as she died already in 1732.

7. I. Barker apparently to Mother Theresa [Lady Lucy Herbert], 14 August 1739, in H. Tayler (ed.), *Lady Nithsdale and Her Family* (London, 1939), pp. 239–40.

8. The medieval tradition of the healing holy kingship (especially for the King's evil), aptly illustrated by Marc Bloch in *The Royal Touch. Sacred Monarchy and Scrofula in England and France*, translated by J. E. Anderson (London: Routledge, 1973), was alive and well when Queen Anne was in the process of healing the poor. To the Duchess of Marlborough, Kensington, April 29, 1706, in B. C. Brown, *Queen Anne, The Letters and Diplomatic Instructions of Queen Anne* (London: Cassell, 1968), p. 185. On late medieval kingship, see also E. H. Kantorowicz, *The King's Two Bodies. A Study in Mediaeval Political Theology* (Princeton: Princeton University Press, 1957/1981); M. Kaartinen, *Religious Life and English Culture in the Reformation* (Basingstoke and New York: Palgrave, 2002).

9. King, *Jane Barker*, pp. 69–76. On her interest in anatomy, pp. 84–96. Barker wrote a long poem on anatomy, published in *Poetical Recreations Consisting of Original Poems, Songs, Odes, &c.* (London, 1688).

10. Guy, *A Select Number of Schirrhus and Cancerous Cases*, pp. 25–6, 37.

11. For a modern biography, see R. Perry, *The Celebrated Mary Astell. An Early English Feminist* (Chicago and London: The University of Chicago Press, 1986).

12. Astell kept her illness so well guarded that we know about it almost exclusively because of George Ballard, who wrote about it in his *Memoirs of Several Ladies of Great Britain* (1752); this account was repeated in other collections. Only thus, and clearly against her wishes, did Astell's breast cancer become public knowledge. G. Ballard, *Memoirs of Several Ladies of Great Britain, who have been Celebrated for their Writings or Skill in the Learned Languages Arts and Sciences* (Oxford, 1752), pp. 445–9. See also *Biographium Fæmineum. The Female Worthies: or, Memoirs of the Most Illustrious Ladies, of All Ages and Nations*, vol. 1 (London, 1766). This account is also partly cited in P. Crawford and L. Gowing, *Women's Worlds in Seventeenth-Century England. A Sourcebook* (London and New York: Routledge, 2000), pp. 27–8; See also Epstein, 'Writing the Unspeakable', p. 155.

13. Ballard, *Memoirs of Several Ladies*, p. 459; see also Perry, *The Celebrated Mary Astell*, pp. 318–319, Crawford and Gowing, *Women's Worlds*, p. 28.

14. L. Whaley, *Women and the Practice of Medical Care in Early Modern Europe, 1400–1800* (Basingstoke and New York: Palgrave, 2011); S. Broomhall, *Women's Medical Work in Early Modern France* (Manchester: Manchester University Press, 2004); on self-medication, Porter and Porter, *Patient's Progress*, pp. 33–52, on women as healers, pp. 177–8; Beier, *Sufferers & Healers*, pp. 216, 241; Wear, *Knowledge and Practice*, pp. 21–2; R. R. O'Day, 'Tudor and Stuart Women: Their Lives through their Letters', in J. Daybell (ed.) *Early Modern Women's Letter Writing, 1450–1700* (Basingstoke and New York: Palgrave), pp. 127–42; W. Kerwin, *Beyond the Body. The Boundaries of Medicine and English Renaissance Drama* (Amherst and Boston, MA: University of Massachusetts Press, 2005), pp. 68–82. On Lady Grace Mildmay, see L. Pollock, *With Faith and*

Physic. The Life of a Tudor Gentlewoman. Lady Grace Mildmay 1552–1620 (New York: St Martin's Press, 1993); R. M. Warnicke, 'Lady Mildmay's Journal: A Study in Autobiography and Meditation in Reformation England', *Sixteenth Century Journal*, 20:1 (1989), pp. 55–68; S. C. Seelig, *Autobiography and Gender in Early Modern Literature. Reading Women's Lives, 1600–1680* (Cambridge: Cambridge University Press, 2006), p. 26. On Lady Margaret Hoby, see J. Moody (ed.), *The Private Life of an Elizabethan Lady. The Diary of Lady Margaret Hoby 1599–1605* (Sutton: Stroud, 1998); On Lady Anne Halkett, A. Halkett, *The Autobiography of Anne Lady Halkett* (London: Camden Society, 1875); O'Day, *The Professions*, p. 214; Fissell, *Vernacular Bodies*, p. 108; E. Grey, *A Choice Manual of Rare and Select Secrets in Physick and Chyrurgery* (London, 1687), pp. 44–6, 523–8, 103–4, 118–9.

15. Perry, *Colonizing the Breast*, p. 234.
16. Anon., *An Account*, pp. 27–8; Hill, *Plain and Useful Directions*, p. 3. For this medication in use, ibid., p. 28. See also O'Day, *The Professions*, p. 209.
17. Hannah Murray of Stratford, taken from her own mouth the 12th of July, 1745. Gentlemen of the Faculty, *The Medical Museum*, vol. 1, pp. 84–5.
18. Wear, *Knowledge and Practice*, pp. 55–67. On the open world of medicine, see Porter & Porter, *Patient's Progress*, pp. 26–9.
19. On cancer medications, see also M. J. O'Dowd, *The History of Medications for Women. Materia Medica Woman* (New York and London: The Parthenon Publishing Group, 2001), p. 127.
20. Anon, *Treasure of Pore Men* (London, 1526), p. 28; same recipe also on p. 40.
21. A. T., *A Rich Storehouse, or Treasurie for the Diseased Wherein are Many Approued Medicines for Diuers and Sundry Diseases* (London, 1631), p. 87.
22. Anon., *A Book of Fruits & Flowers. Shewing the Nature and Use of them, Either for Meat or Medicine* (London, 1653), p. 18.
23. H. Woolley, *The Gentlewomans Companion; or, A Guide to the Female Sex Containing Directions of Behaviour, in All Places, Companies, Relations, and Conditions, from their Childhood Down to Old Age* (London, 1673), p. 170.
24. H. Woolley, *The Accomplish'd Lady's Delight in Preserving, Physick, Beautifying, and Cookery* (London, 1675), p.155.
25. C. Brooks, *The Complete English Cook; or, Prudent Housewife. Being an Entire New Collection of the Most Genteel, yet Least Expensive Receipts in Every Branch of Cookery and Good Housewifery* (London, [*c.* 1770]), p. 114.
26. The celandine referred to here was probably the *Chelidonium majus* (tetter-wort or swallow-wort), the bright yellow latex (produced when the stem is broken) of which was used for example to treat eye problems. OED. Interestingly, *Chelidonium majus* belongs to the *Papaveraceae* family and is related to the poppy. *Chelidonium majus* is presently used in homeopathy, with very similar indications.
27. Ann, Countess of Coventry possessed at least 'Harvy's Physitian', which was probably Gideon Harvey's *Family Physician, and the House Apothecary*. S. Pennell, 'Introduction', in N. Glaisyer and S. Pennell (eds) *Didactic Literature in England 1500–1800. Expertise Constructed* (Aldershot and Burlington, VT: Ashgate, 2003), pp. 1–18. Woolley also recommended a medicine based on leeks, yarrow and white wine. Woolley, *The Accomplish'd Lady's Delight*, p. 136, and a green ointment on p. 148. Other medications for cancers and sores: Anon., *A Booke of Soueraigne Approued Medicines and Remedies as Well for Sundry Diseases Within the Body as Also for All Sores, Woundes, Goutes, and Other Griefes Whatsoeuer, That Greeue or Moleste the Bodye, or any Parte Thereof* (Lon-

don, 1577), ff. A8v; C4r–v; A.T., *A Rich Storehouse*, pp. 83, 84, 87; *A Closet for Ladies and Gentlewomen, or, The Art of Preserving, Conserving, and Candying*, 1614, pp. 167, 175; Gentleman of the Faculty, *Every Lady her own Physician*, pp. 61–2, 71–2, lists a significant number of recipes for cancer. E. Smith, *The Complete Housewife or, Accomplished Gentlewoman's Companion. Being a Collection of Upwards of Seven Hundred of the Most Approved Receipts*, 18th edn (London, 1773), pp. 322–3 lists popular remedies, one of which, a lozenge, was made of 'the powder of crab's-claws' and rosewater. Ibid., p. 323. See also *Trotula*, p. 102.

28. On recipe collections, see Leong and Pennell, 'Recipe Collections'.

29. Household and medical recipes, Wellcome Library, MSL. MS. 2.

30. The poultice, Household and medical recipes, Wellcome Library, MSL. MS. 2, f. 36; Chiselden's recipe advises the patient to boil wormwood, St. John's wort, rosemary, scordium [Water-Germander, lat. *Teucrium Scordium*], and chamomile in water, then to drain and finally mix the liquid with alcohol, for example 'good french Brandy'. It is used in a dressing which is laid on the ulcer, filling the hole with layers of the warm liquid, and changing the dressing each morning and evening. Household and medical recipes, Wellcome Library, MSL. MS. 2, f. 182.

31. Recipe Collection, Wellcome Library, MS 2323. Mary Eyton has signed on the cover 'Mary Eyton her book'. She is most likely to have owned the book in the 1690s, since a date of 19 December 1691 is marked on the cover. We cannot tell for certain whether Amy Eyton owned the book before or after Mary, but the first folio of the manuscript declares, 'Amy Eyton her Book pris 2 s'. The mention of the price suggests Amy may have been the first owner of the book, which would give the collection a significantly longer lifespan. Elsewhere in the collection, Sarah Justice has inscribed her name as well. The last date given in the collection is 1738.

32. Arscott Family Physical Receipts, Wellcome MS 981. See also Coates, 'Female Disorders', pp. 81–5. One very common and interesting medication for cancer was made of corns of horses: 'Take ye Cornes of ye fore leggs of a stone Hors or gelding dye ym in an oven Carefully & Beat ym to a Powder & sift ym to a fine Powder take 2 grains with half ye grantelic of Powder of Mace & 2 or 3 spoonfulls of sack & night & morning ye first & last thing take 2 or 3 spoonfulls of ye Juce of Elder leaves as yo find it purg take it once in 10 days yo must be Bloodied once or twise in 5 or 6 wecks take this medicine 3 wecks togather yn rest a while yn repeating of twise yo will find ye benifit off it, yo must Eat nor drink any thing yo Must purg before yo take ye medicin with Elder, if in winter it must be surup of ye Iuce of ye leaves. Recipe Collection, Wellcome Library, MS 2323, f. 106v. Arscott Family Physical Receipts, Wellcome MS 981, f. 162 includes this recipe from two sources: Mrs Fuller and Dr Dobbs from Dublin. The horse warts or corns do come up in the literature every now and then. They are recommended for example for cancers in a family medical book, *The Family Pocket-Book* ([*c.* 1762]), f. 145, and Richard Guy mentions that a surgeon had prescribed it to a patient of his. – Guy, *Practical Observations*, p. 153. John Ball notes that it was a favourite amongst 'empyrical medicines', 'much cried up by many people', but this does not prevent him from listing it among possible medications for cancer. By including the horse warts in his *The Female Physician*, he in a way legitimizes anyone to try them, just in case. See Ball, *The Female Physician*, p. 103. Eliza Smith's best-seller *The Complete Housewife*, p. 322, also listed a variation on the recipe.

33. Arscott Family Physical Receipts, Wellcome MS 981, separate leaf in front of volume, nr 2. (author anonymous)

34. Ibid., pp. 160–1.
35. Ibid., p. 167.
36. Ibid., pp. 17, 76, 152, 171.
37. Fissell, *Vernacular Bodies*, pp. 7–8; S. Skedd, 'Women Teachers and the Expansion of Girls' Schooling in England, c. 1760–1820', in B. Hannah and E. Chalus (eds), *Gender in Eighteenth-Century England. Roles, Representations and Responsibilities* (London and New York: Longman, 1997), pp. 101–25; Earle, *A City Full of People*, pp. 28–38.
38. Porter, 'Spreading Medical Enlightenment', pp. 215–6; Fissell, 'Readers, Texts, and Contexts', p. 92. Glaisyer and Pennell suggest that the vernacularization of professional texts, in particular medical texts, undermined the monopoly of the educated medical profession, especially physicians. In other words, vernacular medical texts made the secrets of the professionals available to laymen. Glaisyer and Pennell, 'Introduction', p. 11. An excellent example of such a text was Lewis Mansey's commonsensical account, which gives a summary of contemporary understanding of breast cancer. It was intended for all kinds of readers. Mansey, *The Practical Physician*. See also Porter and Porter, *Patient's Progress*, p. 6. This is undoubtedly true; but there is another side to the story. As we have seen, medical knowledge was always shared; early modern medicine was not yet a specialized topic as such. A great number of medical books were published for everyone to read, and after the coming of the printing press most medical books were published in English. Webster counted that 238 medical books were published in England between 1640 and 1660 alone, and of these publications only 31 were in Latin. Cited in Wear, *Knowledge and Practice*, p. 41. On popular medical books as part of the medical marketplace, see M. E. Fissell: 'The Marketplace of Print', in Jenner and Wallis (eds), *Medicine and the Market*, pp. 108–32. But it is also true that popular literature and advice books, such as I. Moore, *The Useful and Entertaining Family Miscellany: Containing the Complete English Housekeeper's Companion* (London, 1766), pp. 71–2, included advice on cancer and its treatments copied from learned medical books, and thus transmitted accepted professional medical information on this illness in a more accessible form than some treatises primarily intended for the medical faculty. Vernacular medical texts did not necessarily reach the poor, as Paul Slack has pointed out, but they reflect 'some of the medical problems and attitudes', and are thus useful in exploring the information available to laymen. P. Slack, 'Mirrors of Health and Treasures of Poor Men: The Uses of the Vernacular Medical Literature of Tudor England', in C. Webster (ed.) *Health, Medicine and Mortality in the Sixteenth Century* (Cambridge: Cambridge University Press, 1979), pp. 237–73. Andrew Wear notes that the term 'popular' in 'popular books' did not really mean a text for everyone: they were for the literate. Wear, 'The Popularization of Medicine', pp.17–18.
39. Fissell, *Vernacular Bodies*, p. 1; P. Borsay, *The English Urban Renaissance. Culture and Society in the Provincial Town 1660–1770* (Oxford: Clarendon, 2003), p. 131; Berry, *Gender, Society and Print Culture*, p. 125.
40. According to Mary Fissell, that this has been suggested by Monica Green, Helen King, Patricia Crawford and Robert Martenson. See Fissell, *Vernacular Bodies*, p. 7. Fissell argues that in this literature the female body became a battleground: 'Women's bodies were sites of contest, places that people argued about and through which they tried to construct themselves as authoritative'. Ibid., pp. 12–13. Her study of the female body in vernacular literature stresses the importance of oral information in the passing on of information about the body: everyone heard jokes and sang ballads, p. 2. Medical as well as surgical information was passed from one person to another. Even information about

physicians and surgeons specializing in breast problems was passed on, as we will soon see. It must also be kept in mind that in the eighteenth century women as well as men eagerly attended scientific lectures, suggesting that women too were interested in learning about and understanding their world. In early nineteenth-century York, Jane Ewbank heard lectures on astronomy, science and galvanism; M. Hallett and J. Rendall, 'Preface', in Hallett and Rendall (eds) *Eighteenth-Century York: Culture, Space and Society* (York: Borthwick Institute of Historical Research, University of York, 2003), pp. ix–x. Medical and surgical societies existed along with other specialized societies, but women were probably not members of these. Borsay, *The English Urban Renaissance*, p. 136; P. Borsay, 'Politeness and Elegance: The Cultural Re-Fashioning of Eighteenth-Century York', in Hallett and Rendall (eds), *Eighteenth-Century York*, pp. 1–12. On clubs and societies, see P. Clark, *British Clubs and Societies 1580–1800. The Origins of an Associational World* (Oxford and New York: Oxford University Press, 2000).

41. Borsay, *The English Urban Renaissance*, pp. 133–4; Porter and Porter, *Patient's Progress*, pp. 203–2.

42. J. Bell, *A New Catalogue of Bell's Circulating Library, Consisting of Above Fifty Thousand Volumes* (London, 1778), cover.

43. Ibid., p. 11.

44. Ibid., p. 22.

45. Ibid., pp. 163–73.

46. *A Catalogue of R. Fisher's Circulating Library, in the High-Bridge, Newcastle* (Newcastle, 1791), pp. 135, 137.

47. Stories of miraculous healings of cancer were available from ancient sources. Augustine's remarks on the miracle of Innocentia, who was miraculously cured of breast cancer, were apparently well-known in the seventeenth century if not later. H. L'Estrange, *The Alliance of Divine Offices, Exhibiting All the Liturgies of the Church of England Since the Reformation* (London, 1659), p. 246. In North America, I. Mather, *An Essay for the Recording of Illustrious Providences Wherein an Account is Given of Many Remarkable and Very Memorable Events which have Hapned this Last Age, Especially in New-England* (Boston, MA, 1684), p. 272, also discussed the case and located the legend in Augustine, *De civitate dei*, book 22, chapter 8. I have used the 1610 edn, where Innocentia's legend is found on pp. 884–5. See also de Moulin, *A Short History of Breast Cancer*, p. 12.

48. Discussed also in de Moulin, *A Short History of Breast Cancer*, pp. 24–6; R. Kleinman, *Anne of Austria. Queen of France* (Columbus, OH: Ohio State University Press, 1985), pp. 283–6.

49. For example *The Edinburgh Repository for Polite Literature, Consisting of Elegant, Instructive, and Entertaining Extracts* (Edinburgh, 1793), pp. 381–2.

50. M. Barber, *Poems on Several Occasions* (London, 1734), p. 76.

51. Gregory of Nyssa, *Life of St Macrina*, 992a–992b. St Macrina died in 379. She is also briefly mentioned in V. Burrus, *The Sex Lives of Saints: An Erotics of Ancient Hagiography* (Philadelphia, PA: University of Pennsylvania Press, 2004), p. 75 and Yalom, *A History of the Breast*, p. 31; de Moulin, *A Short History of Breast Cancer*, p. 12. On the healing powers of feminine tears in medieval tradition, see L. M. Bishop, *Words, Stones, & Herbs. The Healing Word in Medieval and Early Modern England* (Syracuse, NY: Syracuse University Press, 2007), p. 144.

52. King, *Hippocrates' Woman*, p. 47.

53. *Trotula*, p. 65.

54. S. Sontag, *Illness as Metaphor and AIDS and Its Metaphors* (London: Penguin 1978/2002), pp. 18, 20. Sontag famously observes that leukaemia, a cancer without tumours, is romanticized in a way comparable to the romantic disease of the nineteenth century, tuberculosis – it consumes the young and the beautiful. Otherwise cancer holds no romantic connotations whatsoever, p. 51. For critical readings of Sontag, see for example B. Clow, 'Who's Afraid of Susan Sontag? or, the Myths and Metaphors of Cancer Reconsidered', *Social History of Medicine*, 14:2 (2001), pp. 293–312.

55. Ballard, *Memoirs*, p. 459; also cited in Crawford and Gowing, *Women's Worlds*, pp. 27–8.

56. Ballard, *Memoirs*, p. 459; Perry, *The Celebrated Mary Astell*, p. 320.

57. Ballard, *Memoirs*, p. 459; Perry, *The Celebrated Mary Astell*, p. 320; Crawford and Gowing, *Women's Worlds*, p. 28.

58. Guy, *An Essay*, p. 27.

59. Ibid., p. 28.

60. Cf. Fissell, *Vernacular Bodies*, p. 61.

61. Tissot, *The Lady's Physician*, pp. 1–2.

62. *Modern Family Physician*, p. 220.

63. Guy, *Practical Observations*, p. 56.

64. David E. Shuttleton's interpretation of Mary Chandler's poem *Description of Bath* suggests that the author calls on the ladies to escape the male gazes of the spa with her: 'Chandler's muse actively calls her implied women readers to fly with her away from 'this enchanting Place', whilst pointing towards 'a safe Retreat' in Leake's bookshop and circulating library'. D. E. Shuttleton, 'Mary Chandler's *Description of Bath* (1733): A Tradeswoman Poet of Georgian Urban Renaissance', in Sweet and Lane (eds) *Women and Urban Life*, pp. 173–94.

65. Kaartinen, 'Women Patients'.

66. It would be pointless to list here all the numerous cases in which friends were consulted but in Hill, *Cases in Surgery*, p. 22, it at least seems quite possible that friends were informed of the melancholy diagnosis before the patient.

67. Burrows, *A New Practical Essay on Cancers*, pp. 91–2.

68. Morgan, Casebook, 1714–1747, Wellcome MS 3631, f. 64.

69. M. Kaartinen, '"Pray, Dr, is there Reason to Fear a Cancer?" Fear of Breast Cancer in Early Modern Britain', in J. Liliequist (ed.), *A History of Emotions, 1200–1800* (London: Pickering & Chatto, 2012), pp. 153–66.

70. Porter and Porter, *Patient's Progress*, pp. 53–69; O'Day, *The Professions*, pp. 183–6, 222.

71. Guy, *Practical Observations*, p. 87.

72. O'Day, *The Professions*, p. 193.

73. Female surgeons were a rarity. Margaret Pelling's study of Norwich reveals that the town had one female surgeon, but that one-third of all medical practitioners were female – and this figure does not include midwives. Pelling, *The Common Lot*, pp. 86; 226–7; M. Pelling and C. Webster, 'Medical Practitioners', in C. Webster, *Health, Medicine and Mortality in the Sixteenth Century* (Cambridge: Cambridge University Press, 1979), pp. 165–235 Beier, *Sufferers & Healers*, pp. 28, 218–24; Porter and Porter, *Patient's Progress*, p. 177; P. K. Wilson, 'Acquiring Surgical Know-How. Occupational and Lay Instruction in Early Eighteenth-Century London', in R. Porter (ed.) *The Popularization of Medicine 1650–1850* (London and New York: Routledge, 1992), pp. 42–71; O'Day, *The Professions*, pp. 214, 219–220; Wear, *Knowledge and Practice*, p. 211; Seelig, *Autobiography and Gender*, p. 26; Broomhall, 'Medicine and Women', pp. 255–61; Katritzky, *Women, Medi-*

cine and Theatre, pp. 139, 142–3, 164. See also Bishop, *Words, Stones, and Herbs*, pp. 130–52, and on women healers in Antiquity, Nutton, *Ancient Medicine*, pp. 100–2, 198.

74. Berry, *Gender, Society and Print Culture*, p. 128. On irregular practitioners of medicine and their methods, Porter and Porter, *Patient's Progress*, pp. 96–102, and on the use of their services, pp. 103–8.

75. Katritzky, *Women, Medicine and Theatre*, passim, and D. Gentilcore, *Medical Charlatanism in Early Modern Italy* (Oxford and New York: Oxford University Press, 2006), on surgical specialists especially see pp. 181–96, on the performances, pp. 310–34, are thorough studies of these professions in Europe. They do not mention any performances on cancers, suggesting that these were not very common.

76. Glanvill, *Essays*, p. 55. Also in Glanvill, *Saducismus Triumphatus*, p. 91. These repeat what is said in Greatrakes's treatise Dean Rust's certificate. See V. Greatrakes, *A Brief Account of Mr Valentine Greatrakss, and Divers of the Strange Cures By Him Lately Performed* (London, 1666). For a comprehensive study on Greatrakes, see Nurminen, 'Anatomiaa ja ihmetekoja', 2012. For more on Greatrakes, see E. Duffy, 'Valentine Greatrakes, the Irish Stroker: Miracles, Science and Orthodoxy in Restoration England' in K. Robbins (ed.), *Religion and Humanism: Papers Read at the Eighteenth Summer Meeting and the Nineteenth Winter Meeting of the Ecclesiastical History Society* (Oxford: Blackwell, 1981), pp. 251–173; B. B. Kaplan, 'Greatrakes the Stroker: The Interpretations of His Contemporaries', *Isis*, 73:2 (1982), pp. 178–185; A. Marshall, 'The Westminster Magistrate and the Irish Stroker: Sir Edmund Godfrey and Valentine Greatrakes, Some Unpublished Correspondence', *Historical Journal*, 40:2 (1997), pp. 499–505. Also noted by Wear, *Knowledge & Practice*, p. 429; Porter and Porter: *Patient's Progress*, p. 27.

77. Marshall, 'The Westminster Magistrate', p. 500.

78. H. Stubbe, *The Miraculous Conformist, or, An Account of Severall Marvailous Cures Performed by the Stroking of the Hands of Mr. Valentine Greatarick with a Physicall Discourse Thereupon* (Oxford, 1666), p. 3.

79. Greatrakes, *A Brief Account*, pp. 84–5. It also includes testimony of the healing of a sore breast 'which had several holes in it for the space of 14 weeks', on p. 86.

80. Stubbe, *The Miraculous Conformist*, p. 3.

81. D. Defoe, *The Compleat Mendicant: or, Unhappy Beggar, being The Life of an Unfortunate Gentleman* (London, 1699), pp. 24–5.

82. Rowley, *A Treatise on the Management of Female Breasts*, p. 71; he continues against quacks, pp. 72–3.

83. Bell, *A System of Surgery*, vol. 5, p. 173.

84. Hill, *Cases in Surgery*, p. 67. She was operated but it did not prove successful.

85. She reported her history to Samuel Young, the surgeon who eventually published her case in 1815. Young notes that he is publishing Mrs Jenning's own statement; to corroborate his words, her story is given in quotation marks in his text, giving us cause to believe his words. There is of course no evidence of the account being of her own writing or speech, but actually we have no reason to believe Young was lying. It is probable that he considered that for medical reasons it might be informative for the reader to receive this account as he had had it, at first hand from Mrs Jennings, who, he says, had wanted her name to be made public. Young, *Minutes*, p. 127.

86. Ibid., pp 33–4.

87. Ibid.

88. Wiseman, *Eight Chirurgical Treatises*, p. 175.

89. I have discussed this in 'Women Patients'.

90. Nooth, *Observations*, p. 67.

91. Burrows, *A New Practical Essay on Cancers*, p. 95.

92. For places of help, see Kaartinen, 'Women Patients'.

93. Dionis, *A Course of Chirurgical Operations*, p. 253.

94. Buchan, *Domestic Medicine*, p. 602. The exact same wording can be found in Culpeper, *Culpeper's English Physician*, p. 181.

95. Culpeper, *Culpeper's English Physician*, p. 182.

96. Wear, *Knowledge and Practice*, pp. 236, 239.

97. Duncan, *Medical Cases*, p. 111.

98. Gooch, *The Chirurgical Works*, vol. 3, p. 185.

99. Below I discuss others, as well as yet another case: Fearon, *A Treatise on Cancers*, 1790, pp. 199–200.

100. Fearon mentions that this had occurred some eight years earlier; his book was published in 1790.

101. Fearon, *A Treatise on Cancers*, p. 141.

102. Ibid., pp. 141–2.

103. Ibid., p. 142.

104. Ibid., pp. 145–6.

105. Ibid., pp.147–8. His other cases: a widow waited for six months before consenting to an operation; she survived the operation, carried out in 1781, and was still alive when Fearon wrote his book; pp. 150–1.

106. Ibid., pp. 158–9.

107. Duncan, *Medical Cases*, p. 114.

108. This was normal practice; for more on it see Porter & Porter, *Patient's Progress*, pp. 79–81. Joseph Binns for example had a patient who left his care and who entrusted her life to a chemist, who promised to cure her breast cancer as he had boasted to have cured 'those that have been 10 times worse'. She died in only 10 days. BL, Sloane 153, ff. 244–5; see also Beier, *Sufferers & Healers*, p. 53.

109. Ewart, *The History of Two Cases of Ulcerated Cancer of the Mamma*, p. 30.

110. Fearon, *A Treatise on Cancers*, pp. 66–7.

111. Ibid., pp. 156.

112. Ibid., pp. 168–9.

113. Guy, *Practical Observations*, pp. 168–9.

114. Wiseman, *Eight Chirurgical Treatises*, p. 168.

115. Rowley, *Seventy Four Select Cases*, p. 8.

116. Duden, *The Woman Beneath the Skin*, p. 62; Fissell, *Patients, Power, and the Poor*, pp. 68–70. See also Fissell, 'Readers, Texts, and Contexts', p. 92; Fissell: 'The Marketplace of Print'.

117. I believe I have been able to identify her (the location, her age and the time of the birth of her son in the records match the account) in http://www.familysearch.org. She was Mary Jennings, née Curtis, from Harlington, Bedfordshire. Mary Curtis was born *circa* 1760 in Harlington, and married John Wingate Jennings. The couple had two children: John, who died in 1793 at the age of ten, and Elizabeth, who was born in March, six months before John's death. Elizabeth probably survived childhood, as there is a marriage of an Elizabeth Jennings to George Pearse in Harlington in 1819. Mrs Jennings must have been a notable person in Harlington, since her husband, John Wingate Jennings (senior) seems to have been in possession of the considerable Wingate estate there. (http://www.british-history.ac.uk/report.asp?compid=42450) There was grief in

Mrs Jennings's life. As said, she lost her son John in 1793. His death must have been a blow to her – it was not, after all, an everyday occasion to lose a child of that age. One might expect a younger child to die of a disease, but ten-year-olds usually died only from aggressive epidemics or through an accident. She lost her husband in 1810; he was buried March 7th. As mentioned, her lump started to grow at that time – it is possible that she remembered the lump so well because of her husband's simultaneous death, and that she considered her grief to have been the origin of the disease.

118. Young, *Minutes*, pp. 133–4.
119. Ibid., p. 134.
120. Ibid.
121. Ibid., pp. 134–5.
122. Ibid., p. 135. Italics original.
123. Ibid.
124. Ibid., p. 127.
125. I would like to entertain hope that she lived to see her probably only child Elizabeth marry in 1819, but I have found no record of the date of her death, and it remains unclear.
126. Coltman, *An Address to the Public*, pp. 21–4.
127. Latta, *A Practical System of Surgery*, vol. 2, p. 510.
128. Ibid., p. 511.
129. Ibid., p. 533.
130. Guillemeau, *A Worthy Treatise*, p. 57.
131. Mansey, *The Practical Physician*, p. 373.
132. Parkinson, *Medical Admonitions*, p. 469.
133. Ibid.
134. Ibid., pp. 469–70.
135. Ibid., p. 471.
136. Ibid., pp. 471–2.
137. In about 1698 Mrs. Woeden's tumour became very painful, and she had it operated on six months later. This is relatively early. Her surgeon William Cowper had intended to mention the time she had had a tumour but apparently forgot to add the date in his manuscript – or perhaps he forgot to ask her again if it had slipped his mind. There is a blank in the space of the date intended. Cowper, Surgical operations, BL, Sloane MS 3409, f. 10v.
138. Ibid., f. 4v.
139. Mustow, Commonplace book, BL, Sloane MS 2117, f. 160.
140. Ibid.
141. Nooth, *Observations*, p. 61.
142. Guy, *An Essay*, p. 29.
143. Hill, *Cases in Surgery*, pp. 21–2.
144. *Medical Observations and Inquiries*, vol. 4, p. 362.
145. She was in such pain that she ground her teeth so forcefully that Nicolson wrote 'he really thought her teeth must have been ground to pieces'. Ibid., pp. 364–6.
146. Hunter, *The Case Books*, pp. 10–11.
147. Ibid., p. 40–1, 442
148. This text is printed in Burney, *The Journals and Letters*, vol. 6, pp. 596–616; and partly in Porter & Porter, *In Sickness and in Health*, pp. 107–10; it discussed in several contexts, including A. R. Moore, 'Preanesthetic Mastectomy: A Patient's Experience', *Surgery* 83:2 (1978), pp. 200–205; de Moulin, *A Short History of Breast Cancer*, pp. 55–6; Epstein,

'Writing the Unspeakable'; Dally, *Women under the Knife*, pp. 104–109; Johannisson, *Kroppens tunna skal*, p. 80; Yalom, *History of the Breast*, pp. 221–5; K. Torney, 'Fanny Burney's Mastectomy', *Meridian* 10:2 (1991), pp. 79–85, offers a psychoanalytical interpretation of the text. See also Morris, *The Culture of Pain*, p. 63; Richter, *Missing the Breast*, pp. 77–9.

149. Burney, *The Journals and Letters*, vol. 6, pp. 596–616, esp. 613. Epstein, 'Writing the Unspeakable', pp. 137, 140.

150. Burney, *Journals and Letters*, vol. 6, pp. 806–8.

151. Ibid., pp. 643, 649.

152. Ibid., p.613 and n. 35.

153. Kay Torney notes, quite correctly, that Burney's text is not a conventional letter. It lacks much and is far too long to be an ordinary letter. Torney, 'Fanny Burney's Mastectomy', p. 80. Julia Epstein notes that it is 'part medico-surgical treatise and part sentimental fiction'. Epstein argues further: 'While its wealth of detail makes it a significant document in the history of surgical technique, its intimate confessions and elaborately fictive staging, persona-building, and framing make it likewise a powerful and courageous work of literature in which the imagination confronts and translates the body'. Epstein, 'Writing the Unspeakable', p. 131. As said, it was written over an extensive length of time, at least months, and edited; but, importantly, this does not mean that we should not discuss it as an account of Madame D'Arblay's *experience* of her ordeal. Naturally, it cannot be read as an immediate reaction to her experience; clearly, she was also creating the experience as she relived it through in writing, but this is the problem we historians always face when reading our sources: what indeed is the message conveyed? For our purposes, the letter does not need to be true – what would 'true' be in a case like this? – in the most literal sense of the word, since we can believe it reflects what she conceptualized or wanted to conceptualize as her experience nine months after the operation. I believe that we can well use this letter as autobiographical writing, as evidence of the ways in which she construed herself before, during and even after the operation.

154. Burney, *Journals and Letters*, vol. 6, p. 599.

155. Ibid., p. 600.

156. Ibid.

157. Ibid.

158. Ibid., p. 601.

159. Ibid., p. 602.

160. Ibid.

161. Ibid.

162. Ibid., p. 603.

163. Later, Fanny Burney tells us, she was actually told that Dubois had no longer considered an operation a good idea; he had thought that her cancer was 'already internally declared', which meant that she would inevitably suffer a horrible death, and an operation would merely add to her sufferings. Larrey, regardless of this opinion, decided to go on with the operation because there was a chance to save her. Ibid., p. 607.

164. Ibid., p. 604.

165. Ibid.

166. Ibid., p. 606.

167. Ibid., pp. 608–9.

168. Ibid., p. 609.

169. Ibid.

170. Ibid., p. 610.

171. Ibid

172. Ibid.

173. Ibid., pp. 610–1.

174. Ibid., p. 611.

175. Ibid., p. 612.

176. Twenty minutes was the ideal – and maximum – time for a safe operation. Latta, *A Practical System of Surgery*, vol. 2, p. 515.

177. Burney, *Journals and Letters*, vol. 6, p. 613.

178. One possible example of such: Dr Hamilton's gentlewoman patient had a lump removed, and after three years, another one from the same spot. She later died of full blown cancer. Shorter, *Women's Bodies*, p. 243.

179. Rowley, *Seventy Four Select Cases*, p. 22.

180. Richard Kay was born in 1716 to the family of a Bury physician. Kay himself followed in his father's footsteps, and began his career by helping his father. In 1743 he left Bury for London to study at Guy's Hospital for a year. When he returned, he was ready to take on his father's patients, who he noted were numerous. R. Kay, *The Diary of Richard Kay, 1716–51 of Baldingstone, Near Bury. A Lancashire Doctor*, ed. W. Brockbank and F. Kenworthy (Manchester: The Chetham Society, 1968), pp. 1, 66.

181. Mrs Driver has otherwise apparently left no mark of her life in the existing records, and we unfortunately do not even know her first name. I am extremely grateful to Rita Hirst of the Rossendale Group for her help on the Driver family. See also Dally, *Women Under the Knife*, p. 6, also mentions the case.

182. Kay, *The Diary*, p. 134.

183. Ibid.

184. Ibid., pp. 134–5.

185. The visit of the 27th took place very late in the evening and it was dark when he rode home. He had a serious accident while on the road: his horse, and he with it, fell from a bridge into a stream, according to his calculations a fall of about 8 feet. Both were miraculously saved. Ibid., pp. 134–5.

186. Ibid., p. 136.

187. Ibid., p. 141–2.

188. Ibid., p. 142.

189. Ibid., p. 146.

190. Ibid., p. 147.

191. Ibid.

192. Ibid., p. 148.

193. Ibid., pp. 149, 151. There were patients who demanded to be operated on twice, with years between the operations. Mrs. Coleman had two operations separated by twelve years. She kept her first lump in a bottle of spirits. She had undergone the experience of extracting a tumour earlier as well. It had been Melmoth Guy's father who had first removed a tumour from her right breast, twelve years before Melmoth set to the task on the left breast. It must be noted that the Guys did not operate, but used caustic methods to 'draw out' the tumour with its roots. Guy, *A Select Number of Schirrhus and Cancerous Cases*, pp. 25–6.

194. Fearon, *A Treatise on Cancers*, p. 152.

195. Ibid.

196. Ibid., p. 154. Fearon's book includes the case of a colleague whom he supervised in performing a second operation on a patient, Mrs. Butcher from Beaconsfield, whose cancer had returned after the first operation. She was corpulent, and thus there was enough skin to heal the wound by the first intention. Even though the operation had been carried out years earlier, she was according to Fearon still alive. Ibid., pp. 164–5. Another one is that of 'a widowed lady' who had her breast removed by an eminent surgeon in the 'old fashion' (by a circular cut), with rather unpleasant consequences. The wound had not healed well, and the site was now occupied by new growth and a large ulcer. She now had another operation, and healed well by the first intention. Ibid., pp. 166–7.
197. Ibid., p. 153.
198. Ibid., p. 154.
199. Ibid., pp. 154–5.
200. Wilmer, *Cases and Remarks in Surgery*, pp. 123–5.
201. Wiseman, *Eight Chirurgical Treatises*, pp. 179–80.
202. Ibid., p. 183 (case on pp. 181–3).

4 'So Frightful to the Very Imagination': Pain, Emotions and Cancer in the Breast

1. F. de Motteville, *Memoirs for the History of Anne of Austria, Wife to Lewis XIII*, vol. 5 (London, 1725), p. 245.
2. Kaartinen, 'Pray Dr'.
3. Ibid.; R. Baxter, *A Breviate of the Life of Margaret, the Daughter of Francis Charlton of Apply in Shropshire, Esq; And Wife of Richard Baxter* (London, 1681), pp. 90–4.
4. For a fuller account of Anna Seward's case, see Kaartinen, 'Pray Dr'; Anna Seward to Reverend R. Sykes, of Foxholes, Yorkshire. Lichfied, April 20, 1794, in A. Seward: *Letters of Anna Seward*, vol. 3, ed. A. Constable (Edinburgh, 1811), pp. 354–61.
5. Turner, *The Art of Surgery*, vol. 1, p. 72.
6. Ibid., pp. 71–3.
7. Nooth, *Observations*, p. 61.
8. Ibid., p. 66.
9. On fear, terror and affrights as causes of melancholy: R. Burton, *Anatomy of Melancholy* (New York: New York Review of Books, 2001), pp. 261–2, 335–339. On melancholy, M. MacDonald, *Mystical Bedlam: Madness, Anxiety and Healing in Seventeenth-Century England* (Cambridge: Cambridge University Press 1981), pp. 150–60. See also Mikkeli, 'A Melancholy Man'; Sánchez, 'Melancholy and Female Illness'.
10. Nooth, *Observations*, p. 61.
11. Ibid.
12. Ibid.
13. Guy, *Practical Observations*, p. 26.
14. Mustow, Commonplace book, BL, Sloane MS 2117, f. 160. See also Rey, *The History of Pain*, p. 67.
15. Dionis, *A Course of Chirurgical Operations*, pp. 249, 250.
16. Ibid., p. 257.
17. Fearon, *A Treatise on Cancers*, p. 6, quoted passage on p. 8.
18. Ibid., pp. 77–8.

19. Guy, *An Essay*, pp. vi–vii. Guy advertised that he had used the poultice on more than a hundred patients with schirruses and cancers in less than two years' time. In his book he presents twelve select cases, of which seven were breast tumours. Ibid., pp. 67–95.
20. Guy, *Practical Observations*, p. xiv.
21. Fearon, *A Treatise on Cancers*, p. 161.
22. Ibid., pp. 161–3. See also cases among those of Burrows: a poor woman refused to be operated on because she 'feared the severity of the operation', and Mary Smith had similar fears. Burrows, *A New Practical Essay on Cancers*, pp. 94–5, 97–8.
23. Rowley, *Seventy Four Select Cases*, p. 6. Italics in the original.
24. Ibid., p. 11.
25. Ibid., p. 13.
26. Young, *Minutes*, p. 4.
27. Nooth, *Observations*, p. 85.
28. Ibid.
29. Ibid., p. 86.
30. Ibid.
31. Guy, *A Select Number of Schirrhus and Cancerous Cases*, pp. 3–4.
32. Nooth, *Observations*, pp. 52–4.
33. Ibid., p. 55.
34. Ibid.
35. Ibid., p. 75.
36. Mustow, Commonplace book BL, Sloane MS 2117, f. 160
37. Stolberg, *Experiencing Illness*, pp. 27–32; Rey, *The History of Pain*, pp. 50–131; E. Scarry, *The Body in Pain: The Making and Unmaking of the World* (Oxford: Oxford University Press, 1987); Morris: *The Culture of Pain*.
38. On pain related to surgery, see Wear, *Knowledge and Practice*, pp. 216, 241–248.
39. Nisbet, *An Inquiry*, pp. 157–8. Fevers, 'the Hectic' often accompanied these last days. Ibid., p. 174. For an example of a patient dying in a convulsion fit, see Norford, *An Essay*, p. 25. In the view of the French physician Le Febure, a patient with hectic fever could be saved from death only by a miracle. *Medical and Philosophical Commentaries*, vol. 4., p. 60.
40. Burrows, *A New Practical Essay on Cancers*, p. 51, also pp. 55–6; See also Sharp, *A Treatise on the Operations of Surgery*, p. 129; van Swieten, *An Abridgement*, pp. 432, 436; Peyrilhe, *Dissertation on Cancerous Diseases*, pp. 8–9; Pearson, *Principles of Surgery*, p. 215; Temple, *Practice of Physic*, pp. 399–400; Wallis, *The Art of Preventing Diseases*, p. 760; Parkinson, *Medical Admonitions*, pp. 467–8; Nayler, *A Cursory View of the Treatment of Ulcers*, pp. 131–2. For a popular text, see for example J. Theobald, *Every man his own physician. Being, a complete collection of efficacious and approved remedies, for every disease incident to the human body* (London, 1764), p. 7. On 'shooting lancinating pains' in cancer, White, *Practical Surgery*, pp. 42–3; *The Edinburgh Practice*, p. 682. Nisbet, *The Clinical Guide*, pp. 149–50, wrote that '[t]he feeling communicated by schirrus in its progress is frequent lancelating [sic] pain darting through the part, uncommon heat and itchiness, as if the part were exposed to fire, and a sense of puncture as if needles were run into it'. In Nisbet, *An Inquiry*, p. 124 (and again on p. 157; on the functions of pain see also pp. 186–7), he reformulates this: 'This pain is of a peculiar kind; it consists, either of sharp lancilating [sic] throbs, of deep shootings, or, in absence of these, of a constant gnawing, or sense of burning heat diffused over it; or of a pricking, like the thrust of needles'. On the types of pains, see Rey, *The History of Pain*, p. 95.
41. Burrows, *A New Practical Essay on Cancers*, pp. 53–4.

42. Ibid., p. 94–5. On Ann James's sufferings, Gentlemen of the Faculty, *The Medical Museum*, vol. 3, pp. 566–7.

43. Anon., *An Account*, pp. 23–4.

44. Dionis, *A Course of Chirurgical Operations*, p. 249.

45. Ball, *The Female Physician*, pp. 86–7. Similar, almost identical, notes, Gentleman of the Faculty, *Every Lady Her Own Physician*, pp. 68–9. Perhaps Ball was the Gentleman of the Faculty? Similar notes were discussed in Part One as well. See Turner, *The Art of Surgery*, vol.1, p. 77; Brookes, *The General Practice of Physic*, pp. 121–2; Buchan, *Domestic Medicine*, pp. 601–2; Culpeper, *Culpeper's English Physician*, p. 181.

46. Ball, *The Female Physician*, p. 85.

47. Justamond, *An Account*, pp. 7–8.

48. Burrows, *A New Practical Essay on Cancers*, p. 97.

49. Gregory, Case Book 1789, Wellcome MS 5939, ff. 82–82v.

50. Ibid.

51. Ibid., pp. 82–4.

52. Ibid., p. 84.

53. Ibid., p. 108.

54. Rose-coloured inflammation of the skin.

55. Gregory, Case Book 1789, Wellcome MS 5939, f. 110.

56. Ibid., p. 111v.

57. Fos 112 and 113 are empty.

58. Barbara A. Hanawalt, *'Of Good and Ill Repute': Gender and Social Control in Medieval England* (New York and Oxford: Oxford University Press, 1998), p. 75.

59. Rowley, *Seventy Four Select Cases*, pp. 7–8.

60. Ewart, *The History of Two Cases of Ulcerated Cancer of the Mamma*, p. 13.

61. Ibid., p. 15.

62. Ibid., p. 17.

63. Ibid., p. 14.

64. Ibid., p. 15.

65. For David Hume, for example, sympathy – which, as Christine Battersby notes, we would term empathy – 'was not itself a passion but [...] lets the other person's miseries and joys affect me as if they were my own'. C. Battersby, 'The Man of Passion: Emotion, Philosophy and Sexual Difference', in P. Gouk and H. Hills (eds) *Representing Emotions. New Connections in the Histories of Art, Music and Medicine* (Aldershot and Burlington, VT: Ashgate, 2005), pp. 139–153.

66. Ewart, *The History of Two Cases of Ulcerated Cancer of the Mamma*, p. 12.

67. Burney, *Journals and Letters*, vol. 6, p. 604; Torney or Epstein, for example, have not found a clear-cut answer to this question: Torney, 'Fanny Burney's Mastectomy', p. 82; Epstein, 'Writing the Unspeakable', p. 144.

68. Burney, *Journals and Letters*, vol. 6, pp. 604–5.

69. Rey, *The History of Pain*, p. 93.

70. Wear, *Knowledge and Practice*, p. 241.

71. Ibid., pp. 246, 248.

72. Burney, *Journals and Letters*, vol. 6, p. 612. On screaming Burney, see also Morris, *The Culture of Pain*, p. 63.

73. Torney, 'Fanny Burney's Mastectomy', p. 81, see also p. 83.

74. Burney, *Journals and Letters*, vol. 6, pp. 612–3.

75. Ibid., p. 614.

76. Scarry, *The Body in Pain*, p. 4.
77. Morris, *The Culture of Pain*, p. 78.
78. To a degree, utter pain can be ahistorical but the historical nature of its expression makes it conveyable to us. The pain and misery caused by breast disease could be depicted as 'almost inexpressible'. Rowley, *Seventy Four Select Cases*, pp. 13–4. Rey argues for an early modern tendency to keep expression of pain at bay. Rey, *The History of Pain*, p. 69.
79. J. Collier, Essays upon Several Moral Subjects, part III. Of pain (London, 1705), p. 24
80. Frances Day's case can be found in Young, *Minutes*, pp. 109–26.
81. Ibid., p. 109.
82. Ibid., pp. 109–10.
83. Ibid.
84. Young, *Minutes*, p. 110.
85. Ibid.
86. Gregory, Case Book 1789, Wellcome MS 5939, f. 84v.
87. Young, Minutes, p. 110.
88. Ibid.
89. Ibid, p. 111.
90. Ibid.
91. One should note here that for example John Ball had recommended that 'mercury is often found serviceable for resolving schirrhous tumours, as well by external, as by internal application; but then it must only be in a benign and incipient scirrhus. Ball, *The Female Physician*, pp. 92–3.
92. Young, *Minutes*, p. 123.
93. I have used www.familysearch.org. I do not in any sense suggest that the results cover all possibilities or indeed are necessarily accurate. An intriguing turn to Frances Day's story appears if we search for her in the records. In Goldington, one Frances Day married a Thomas Smith on 28 November 1814. Is this indeed our Frances, the suffering girl? The evidence is scanty, and it is quite possible that there were two women named Frances Day in Goldington at that time; Day seems not to have been a particularly rare last name in Bedfordshire. But consider this is our Frances Day. She came to Samuel Smith for treatment in September of that year – would she have by the end of November felt so much better that she indeed might have got married? Samuel Young makes no mention of a marriage taking place, but it would not be his place to do so; after all, he does not give any other personal information on Frances Day either.

    But Frances Day was of an appropriate age to marry. She may have been born in 1794 or 1795. The online records do not easily yield much on our Frances Day. I found no female births under that name in Bedford for 1794 or 1795, but in 1794 a girl named Frances was born to Day family in Balsham, Cambridgeshire.

    Thomas and Frances Smith from Bedford seem to have had at least three children. John was born in August 1819, Sarah in October 1821, and Thomas February 1828. One likes to think that Frances Day survived her ordeal, with two breasts or one, had children, and died peacefully in her bed in January 1858. The records tell of the death of a Mrs Frances Smith, who was born in Bedford in 1795, on 11 January 1858. If this woman is indeed our Frances Day, she lived for forty-three years after her case was published by Samuel Young. Mrs Frances Smith died when she was sixty-three years old.
94. Burney, *Journals and Letters*, vol. 6, pp. 612–3.
95. Porter, *Flesh in the Age of Reason*, pp. 274–7, 279, 286.